EMOTIONAL DISORDERS IN
PHYSICALLY ILL PATIENTS

EMOTIONAL DISORDERS IN PHYSICALLY ILL PATIENTS

Edited by

Robert L. Roessler, M.D.
Norman Decker, M.D.

Department of Psychiatry
Baylor College of Medicine
Houston, Texas

HUMAN SCIENCES PRESS,INC.
72 FIFTH AVENUE
NEW YORK, N.Y. 10011

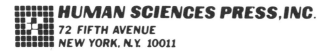

Printed in the United States of America
987654321

Library of Congress Cataloging in Publication Data

Main entry under title:

Emotional disorders in physically ill patients.

   Includes index.
   1. Sick—Psychology. 2. Surgery—Psychological
aspects. 2. Chronic diseases—Psychological
aspects.
I. Roessler, Robert L. II. Decker, Norman.
[DNLM: 1. Disease—psychology.
2. Patients—psychology.
3. Professional-Patient Relations. W 85 E54]
R726.5.E43   1986   616'.0019   85-15120
ISBN 0-89885-254-4

To the memory of our friend and colleague, Dr. Hilde Bruch, who had the courage and strength to extend her meticulous clinical observations, insights and lucid communications to her own disabling and fatal illnesses.

CONTENTS

CONTRIBUTORS

Timothy L. Bayer, M.D.
Assistant Professor of Psychiatry, Baylor College of Medicine
Richard S. Blacher, M.D.
Clinical Professor of Psychiatry, Tufts University School of Medicine
Hilde Bruch, M.D.†
Professor Emeritus of Psychiatry, Baylor College of Medicine
Norman Decker, M.D.
Associate Professor of Clinical Psychiatry and Assistant Professor of Family Medicine, Baylor College of Medicine
Gregory D. Graham, M.D.
Clinical Assistant Professor of Psychiatry, Baylor College of Medicine
Frederick G. Guggenheim, M.D.
Professor and Chairman of Psychiatry, University of Arkansas Medical Sciences
Ismet Karacan, M.D.
Professor of Psychiatry, Baylor College of Medicine
David W. Krueger, M.D.
Clinical Associate Professor of Psychiatry, Baylor College of Medicine
Constance A. Moore, M.D.
Assistant Professor of Psychiatry, Baylor College of Medicine
Robert O. Pasnau, M.D.
Professor of Psychiatry, University of California at Los Angeles
Linda G. Peterson, M.D.
Associate Professor of Psychiatry, University of Massachusetts Medical Center

9

Robert L. Roessler, M.D.
   Professor Emeritus of Psychiatry, Baylor College of Medicine
Chris E. Sermas, M.D.
   Clinical Assistant Professor of Psychiatry, Baylor College of Medicine
James J. Strain, M.D.
   Professor of Psychiatry, Mount Sinai School of Medicine
Avery D. Weisman, M.D.
   Professor of Psychiatry, Harvard Medical School
Robert L. Williams, M.D.
   Professor and Chairman of Psychiatry, Baylor College of Medicine

†*Deceased*

EDITORS' INTRODUCTION

All disease is psychosomatic. Not only does biological dysfunction produce adverse changes in psychological and social function, but adverse psychological and social changes produce change in biological functioning. This book is addressed primarily to physicians but also to resident physicians and fellows, medical students, nurses, social workers, dietitians, occupational and physical therapists—to all professional health care providers who wish to better understand and serve their patients.

The editors and contributors to this book are consultation/liaison (C/L) psychiatrists. The study of biopsychosocial relationships and the application of this knowledge to patient diagnosis and treatment is their professional concern and expertise. They function primarily in hospital settings, where they participate in a broad range of problematic situations in which the interests of patients are at stake. Some of these situations involve psychiatrists' traditional roles of diagnosing and treating psychiatric illnesses, aiding in differential diagnosis, and evaluating patients' competence to give informed consent.

However, C/L psychiatrists typically devote a considerable

proportion of their time to roles that do not fit the usual image of the psychiatrist. These include working with "difficult" patients on medical and surgical services, those who are angry, demanding, clinging, complaining, noncompliant, frightened, confused, and dying. C/L psychiatrists work with such patients to understand why they feel and behave as they do, to relieve their distress, and to expedite their collaboration in their medical care. Such patients often provoke anger, frustration, helplessness, sadness, and grief in those who care for them. Those feelings in care providers can lead to behaviors that adversely affect the quality of patient care: retaliation, rejection, and avoidance. Therefore, C/L psychiatrists also work with care providers to help them understand what is happening to the patient and to them and what can be done to improve the care of the patient. Since the feelings and behavior of patients are often related in part to the feelings and behavior of family members as well, C/L psychiatrists usually work with the family members.

The interests of patients also may be adversely affected by events that do not involve them directly. If nurses are angry at a physician because he has depreciated them, for example, they may express their anger by unconsciously sabotaging or complicating his orders for his patients. The C/L psychiatrist may therefore be involved in group meetings with the medical and nursing staff of an entire unit in efforts to improve staff relationships. Similarly, administrative policies may adversely affect patient care. If there is insufficient recognition of the efforts of care providers, it may result in poor morale that is expressed behaviorally as absenteeism, for example. C/L psychiatrists therefore interact with administrators as well.

C/L psychiatrists also interact frequently and actively with their medical colleagues. They may suggest changes in medications to reduce the likelihood of delirium, emotional distress, and behavioral side effects. They also need to know much about disease generally. They need to know about the natural history of a disease, for example, in order to appreciate the feelings and behavior that are associated with a particular phase of an illness. Such knowledge is often crucial in understanding and treating patients who have suffered severe trauma and those who are chronically ill. Because of these roles the C/L psychiatrist needs to be more broadly informed about medicine than do psychiatrists whose practice is limited to office psychotherapy.

C/L psychiatrists also are involved increasingly in the evaluation and treatment of patients undergoing procedures that have only recently become possible because of technological progress in medicine. These procedures include coronary artery bypass surgery; heart, heart-lung, liver, and kidney transplants; renal dialysis; and cancer therapy. Emotional and behavioral problems are universal in patients undergoing these procedures and in their families as well.

It is clear from this brief review of the roles of C/L psychiatrists that emotional and behavioral problems are present, in greater or lesser degree, in every patient who is physically ill. No single volume can encompass all such problems or encompass their scope, diversity, and complexity. This book is a sampling of some of the more common ones encountered in hospitals and includes discussions of many of the problematic patient behaviors and feelings in which the C/L psychiatrist may be involved. However, primary physicians, house staff, nurses, and other professionals see the patient first. They therefore have the opportunity to identify the problem early. If a C/L psychiatrist does see the patient later, these professionals are primarily instrumental in bringing about changes that the C/L psychiatrist recommends. This book is, therefore, directed primarily to them.

The book is divided into three major sections. The first consists of six chapters on common problems encountered in primary care medicine: crisis on medical wards by Dr. Guggenheim; the causes and treatment of organic brain syndromes by Drs. Roessler and Graham; psychopharmacologic treatment of physically ill patients by Dr. Sermas; problems of pain reviewed by Dr. Bayer; diagnosis and treatment of sleep disorders in medical and surgical patients by Drs. Moore, Karacan, and Williams; the understanding and management of hypochondriasis by Dr. Strain. The second section consists of three chapters on emotional problems in surgical patients. Treatment of the trauma victim is reviewed by Dr. Peterson; the adaptational problems of coronary bypass surgery patients by Dr. Blacher; the problems encountered in obstetrics and gynecology by Dr. Pasnau. The final section focuses on chronic illness. The difficulties of coping with Parkinson's disease are given a sensitive personal perspective by Dr. Hilde Bruch. Dr. Weisman addresses the management of emotional problems of cancer patients. Rehabilitation of chronically disabled adults is reviewed by Dr. Krueger.

All patients' names and other identifiable information have been fictionalized throughout the text. Resemblance to any persons, living or dead, is not intended.

We hope that the reader will come away from this volume with a more sensitive appreciation of what it means to be a patient and a greater appreciation of the importance of his/her own role to the welfare of patients. We also hope that he/she will have a greater understanding of the effects of patients' previous experiences, the effects of the nature of an illness, and the effects of the hospital environment on the feelings and behavior of patients. Most important, we hope that such appreciation and knowledge will help reduce distress and behaviors that complicate and prolong the recovery of patients.

Robert L. Roessler, M.D.
Norman Decker, M.D.

PART I

PROBLEMS IN PRIMARY CARE MEDICINE

Chapter 1

CRISES IN MEDICAL CARE*

Frederick G. Guggenheim

The editors have asked me to discuss crises on medical services. First let us consider what a crisis is. It is a turning point, a challenge to patient, family, and community created by an altered set of circumstances (Schwab, 1968, p. 163). It is a time when things get either better or worse, a time after which an individual or a relationship never remains exactly the same. Another feature of a crisis is that it is a stressful situation perceived as a threat to the self. Crises can come from many causes—birth, death, divorce, graduation, fame, ignominy. I will limit this discussion to crises that occur in a medical setting.

Since I have been around medical services for more than two decades, I have seen many crises, managed some, and learned from at least a few. I will examine here some crises that have had special meanings for me, to see what we can learn together.

Patients' crises, in broad outline, can be grouped into three

*I thank Myron F. Weiner, M.D., and Douglas A. Puryear, M.D., for their thoughtful critiques of earlier versions of this manuscript.

types: impersonal, or biological, medical crises; interpersonal, or sociological crises; and intrapersonal, or psychological crises.

IMPERSONAL CRISES

First let's look at the *impersonal* crisis. Long before any of us swore the Hippocratic oath we were familiar with the exemplar medical crisis, the febrile crisis: The family physician emerges from the child's bedroom, wanly smiles, and tells the concerned parents, "The crisis has passed. The fever has broken. The child will live!" It is a dramatic moment that the child may or may not have been aware of. In modern medicine, impersonal crises are resolved when the lidocaine infusion decreases ventricular excitability of the comatose patient; when the Lown defibrillation paddles are applied to the chest and convert a refractory arrhythmia to normal sinus rhythm; when the infusion of streptokinase gradually opens up the arterial clot so the leg will not have to be amputated after all; when the parenteral haloperidol in the wildly combative post-open-heart surgery patient restores quiet and removes a threat to life.

Psychiatrists usually do not participate directly in these impersonal, biological turning points. Indirectly, of course, we do, since we deal with patients prior to and after the crisis; and we also work with their families and the medical staff "on the front lines" (Guggenheim, 1978). But as consultants, we usually are not with the patient at the time of admission, at discharge/death, or at the moment of biological crisis. Since consultant psychiatrists do not have much experience with impersonal crises, let us leave this behind us and instead look more intently at intrapersonal and interpersonal crises, for they are the heart and soul of consultation liaison psychiatry.

INTERPERSONAL CRISES

Many *interpersonal* crises occur on the medical ward. Some cases are indelibly etched into our memories. My very first psychiatric consultation was certainly that. It began with a real crisis, a turning point, and it was seminal in my later switching from internal medicine to psychiatry. Let me share some details with you.

Case No. 1

Mandy was an eighteen-year-old, single, recent West Coast high school graduate who came to the National Institute of Health (NIH) as part of a study on monozygotic twins discordant for acute leukemia. She had developed her symptoms of leukemia several months after she and her identical twin had graduated from high school. Her twin married, and Mandy had spent that ill-fated summer as a camp counselor. Mandy's leukemia, though active, had not been totally debilitating, and psychologically she seemed to have adjusted to the transcontinental trip to the research hospital in Bethesda and the separation from family.

Then, 5 days after admission a middle-aged minister, dressed in a black suit with a large black hat, arrived unannounced in her room. It was dusk. He looked intently at Mandy and declared: "I've traveled across three states to come to tell you that it is your sin that has brought your leukemia upon you. It's God's will that you die, so I'm here to pray with you for your sins!" At this Mandy blanched, fled her room, and fainted in front of the nurses' station as the black-shrouded ministerial presence stalked out. No apparition, he got on the elevator and was never heard from again.

An emergency psychiatric consultation was requested. Mandy had become psychotic and remained so over the next few days. Chlorpromazine and much attention from the staff led to the resolution of her schizophreniform psychosis. Gradually, all the hallucinated imagery of angels and devils disappeared.

She had never previously been religious or superstitious, but it did seem that she had been multiply cursed. Born with congenital heart disease and frail as a child, she separated voluntarily from her identical twin sister only after puberty. Marriage had parted her from her twin, against her wishes, 2 months prior to the onset of her leukemia symptoms. During a 2-week period while a camp counselor she developed fever, pharyngi-

tis, and petechiae, all leading to a diagnosis of acute lympho-
cytic leukemia. Although neither Mandy nor her family had
sought notoriety, word of her case and her admission to a research hospital for a bone marrow transplant from her healthy
twin apparently had spread, attracting the attention of the
evangelical minister who precipitated Mandy's crisis.

This crisis was readily acknowledged at the nurses' station
and accepted as such by her care givers, who were touched by
her vulnerability. Never willingly alone, she braved months in a
plastic bubble (a life island support system) during experimental bone marrow suppression with the help of nursing staff that
she knew well and the support from her many physicians. Her
goal of getting home (and not in a pine box) was realized 4
months later during a brief remission of her leukemia.

So open was her crisis that all the medical care givers could
respond warmly and openly to Mandy, all the more so as they
learned about the details of her unfortunate life. She allowed
the staff to form an alliance with her and to help her to chase
away her devils. Psychotherapeutic intervention, and disease
remission, allowed her partially to reestablish a lost symbiosis.

An interpersonal turning point is often so painful that the
afflicted individual needs to leave it behind as promptly as possible. Mandy fled, and when that didn't work she fell prostrate,
fainting and psychotic. Our second case demonstrates a different way of dealing with an interpersonal crisis: signing out of
the hospital against medical advice.

Case No. 2

Norman was a seventy-five-year-old white divorced Mid-
western business executive and artist. He had just retired from
his family business after a year of ceremonial good-byes and
honors from his industry. Nine days later he developed acute
left-sided congestive heart failure. He was hospitalized in a coronary care observation unit (CCU). Within 4 days his arrhythmia was corrected, and symptoms of congestive failure abated.
Because of his chronically brittle, labile ways, a psychiatric consultant suggested that the staff pamper and humor him. His

physician ordered a 2-week period of further observation in the private pavilion to rule out the possibility of myocardial infarction.

He was among several patients in the CCU, admitted about the same time, awaiting transfer to less spartan surroundings. He had seemed to be adjusting well to hospitalization. But when a black patient in the CCU was transferred to the private pavilion before he was, Norman became acutely agitated. He felt that no one was paying attention to him; no one cared; no one respected him. Despite the staff's assurances that his not being transferred to the private pavilion as promptly as one of the other patients did not reflect on his personal or social standing in the hospital community, he precipitously signed out of the hospital against medical advice. In this case the staff failed to intervene psychotherapeutically. They did not tell him that he was being kept in the CCU because he was special or that his longer wait was occasioned by the need to make special accommodation for him.

Irritated and petulant, he dressed rapidly and stalked out after he had called a taxi to take him home. As he was unable to locate the elevator amid the CCU maze, the staff had to help him with directions and point him toward the exit. By the time he got home his confusion had cleared, and he no longer felt enraged, although he dwelt on the "insult" for the next few days.

The son of a prominent industrialist, Norman often had been overshadowed by a stunningly beautiful younger sister and a brilliant younger brother. He never had gained successful recognition from his parents in his own mind. He had had difficulty in separating from them and often felt slighted by them. Because of his behavior he often was treated by them as if he were still a child.

Despite his jovial, master-of-ceremonies public appearance, Norman had long felt neglected by family and associates and devalued by them. In the CCU the "challenge" to his self-worth—a black supposedly being given preferential treatment—could not have been predicted by the hospital staff. Clearly, the perceived social put-down had been more of a threat to his sense of self-concept than the possibility of myocardial damage. Threatened by the implied lack of regard by the hospital staff, despite their later solicitations and admonitions, he fled from that painful experience. The confusion that prevented him from finding the elevator was symbolic of the disorganizing effect of the episode.

In the interpersonal crisis the patient often sees others as causing the problem and others as having a solution: protecting and nurturing. The presence of an acute medical illness by itself does not cause the crisis. Rather, it is the conjunction of the stressor, its perception, and its meaning for the patient. More specifically, it is stress plus acute lowering of self-esteem that begins to interfere with resolution of the dilemma. In Virginia Satir's sense, "the self-esteem becomes hooked" (Satir, 1972, p. 59). Therefore, psychological interventions need to focus on both battered body and battered self-esteem. A reading of the relevant dynamics and an opening up of the communication systems allow staff participation, sharing of feelings, and buttressing support.

The turning points of these interpersonal crises may be easy to identify—a terrified scream or an accusatory blast. And at least in these vignettes, psychiatric intervention was not always prompt enough or sufficient to smooth over all facets of the hospitalizations.

INTRAPERSONAL CRISES

Now let us consider an *intrapersonal* crisis. An intrapersonal crisis represents a different type of turning point, for an intrapersonal crisis may be so silent that the medical care givers have no clear idea that it is taking place. The emitted signals are muted, because the individual sees the problem, and often the solution, as coming from within. The degree of suffering may be intense, but psychic disorganization is not a major component, nor is the acute lack of self-esteem.

Intrapersonal crises often come to staff awareness quietly, rather than with a bang, as when the staff requested that we see a patient whose remoteness troubled them: "Can you please see Marie? She seems so quiet. Maybe she's depressed."

Case No. 3

Marie was a seventy-year-old widowed Puerto Rican grandmother. She had been referred to a metropolitan county (charity) hospital from a remote West Texas town because she had presumptive terminal ovarian carcinoma and was financially destitute. With no visitors and from a non-Mexican culture, she seemed to have little in common with any of the Dallas staff or with other patients. She was seen by a psychiatric resident in a routine consultation, in which it was determined that she was only mildly depressed. No specific interventions had been contemplated. She was presented on attending rounds, and as we were turning to walk away, she made a spontaneous, seemingly offhand comment: "One thing I miss most about being here in the hospital is that I can't hear the birds to sing." Her imagery opened up a whole new vista, for she was a poet, a most knowledgeable and creative one. A quiet, shy woman of great culture and sensitivity, over the next week she taught the staff much about Puerto Rico's culture and poetry, its ornithology and its historical traditions.

Her inner poet, always known to her but hidden by her sullen peasant exterior, reacted to the crisis of her hospitalization by increasing emotional isolation. Her escalating remoteness protected her as she lay unappreciated as a person and alone, dying. She had perceived the problem as entirely hers and had seen no solution to her dilemma. Resignation and disengagement had been her answer to the crisis of nonsupportive anonymity.

After the staff had an opportunity to see her anew because of the consultant's therapeutic action with them, she blossomed. The staff felt her warmth and her majesty. Her death 10 days later was not that of a nameless person, and it had several rainbows of hope about it. Psychotherapeutic intervention allowed Marie to develop a series of relationships that recognized her special qualities and buttressed her dignity at a time when biologically she was being stripped of her very being. Her muted tentative gesture, reaching out with a fanciful comment, reminds us that poetry, as well as prose, has a real place in doing consultation work.

Sometimes cases with an intrapersonal crisis also contain an interpersonal crisis, as is exemplified in the next case.

Case No. 4

Nell was a sixty-five-year-old divorced mother, grand-mother, and social activist for Latin-American causes. She had grown up in an upper-middle-class entrepreneurial British family in South America, been assigned to nannies, and then went off to boarding schools. She was graduated from a distinguished college at an early age, successfully reared a family, and at age fifty sought a divorce and began working for an international relief agency. She labored selflessly and devotedly for the Hispanic poor in this country and abroad. She was an idealist and the most articulate, determined planner that any of her friends had ever known.

A convert to commune living at age fifty-eight, Nell was as aggressive and hard-working as ever when at age sixty-four she developed amyotrophic lateral sclerosis (ALS). After several consultations at famed clinics confirmed her own physician's gloomy diagnosis, she made a trip to a megavitamin healer in the South who claimed that his treatment "would have been successful if only [she] hadn't arrived so late." She then settled down to her own dying by dropping her insistence on harsh, idealistic standards for herself and others. Instead, she focused on nourishing the warm relationships that she had developed in her church and changed her priorities over the next year from social activism to personal involvements.

Then Nell became bedbound for a month and needed supplemental oxygen to relieve dyspnea. She was still able to get around her new apartment with a cane or with the help of her live-in housekeeper/companion. In this gradually deteriorating situation, she calmly announced to each of her dear ones that she would no longer see friends and family "for a bit." She then summoned her physician. Mysteriously, he failed to appear— which was aberrant behavior for him in an otherwise solid doctor/patient relationship. She became increasingly depressed as his expected visit failed to materialize. Finally, she became so despondent that she ripped off her nasal oxygen prongs. At last her physician made a home visit. He had a private conversation with her, from which even her companion/housekeeper was excluded. Following their talk, he agreed to admit Nell to a hospital.

The admission physical examination at the hospital was consistent with a frail, energetic woman with ALS, dyspneic without supplemental oxygen, in good spirits and well organized. That evening she told family members that they "need not call" her the next morning but that she would call them, assuring them of her comfort. Several family members remarked that she sounded in good spirits. The next morning a nurse found her dead in bed. No autopsy was performed.

An almost saintly woman, she pronounced the last year of her life as the best and glowed during it. She managed her intrapersonal crisis with growth and added maturity. She saw her problem as her own and realized that most of the solution lay within her. When she first requested her physician to arrange for her terminal admission to a hospital, her mood was bright and confident. But when her physician failed to come to her, she was plunged into an unexpected interpersonal crisis. Suddenly she felt rejected and rejectable. She generalized perceptions of her faltering social network and even began to doubt her worth. With her self-esteem assaulted by her physician's neglect, she wrote a most uncharacteristic letter to a family member—"You now know the worst of me!" She even requested that the second half of a novel she had just finished be destroyed. She became tormented, although her neurological condition changed little during the 2 weeks prior to her death. After she finally was admitted to the hospital, her interpersonal crisis was resolved, so that her last day was peaceful, full of tender concern for family members. A consummate planner, Nell had arranged for her death to occur away from home, so that her devoted housekeeper wouldn't have to blame herself or cope with her dead body.

Nell's brief interpersonal crisis was tumultuous. She ripped off her nasal oxygen several times and finally forced her physician to attend to her. But her prolonged intrapersonal crisis was a silent one, a very alone one. Silent because euthanasia, suicide, or voodoo death are not readily talked about during a patient's life or while a death is pending. Euthanasia laws protect against abuses. Self-willed death, whether chemical or otherwise, except for England's Exit program (Leo, 1980), is little discussed between patients and physicians. Curiously, family planning belongs at both ends of the life spectrum, but the contraceptive part of it is often more readily broached than a patient's terminal self-planning!

Most crises that we witness are shared events and frequently involve others as helpers, failed helpers, or part of the system in crisis. Most people try to, or need to, share at least a part of their crisis. Reaching out during any psychosocial crisis almost always happens, if only transiently or in fantasy. A few individuals do seem to cherish their aloneness, and some crave secrecy, presumaby trying to protect children, grandchildren, servants, and friends. In such instances no phychiatric consultation is requested, no psychiatrist sees the patient, and no medical service intern knows the intimate details of the case when he walks into the room and sees a woman who had a terminal illness, now lying dead.

DISCUSSION

What lessons can we learn from reviewing these cases? Let us first look at the nature of the crisis itself, and then we will review some of the principles of intervention. It seems evident that a turning point may derive from an external source or an internal one.

Among the components of a medical crisis are psychological symptoms. The phenomenology of an individual in a psychosocial medical crisis (France, 1982; Puryear, 1979) may range from perceptual distortion, a sense of disequilibrium and somatic symptoms, to anxiety and/or depression. When a patient first experiences his/her crisis, tensions are experienced along with a pervasive feeling of helplessness. A thinking disorder may evolve that is subtle, or one that is gross with clearly demonstrable confusion. Festinger (1957) has referred to this as cognitive confusion or dissonance; the afflicted person is unable to understand either why situations have occurred or what the event is going to do to him/her. For the patient, both the evaluation of the problem and rational decision-making about it may become impeded. The individual may even lose the ability to predict or to work on the problem anymore. The crisis becomes managed by adjusting coping style to a new reality. After the resolution of a crisis, the perception of crisis abates although the stress itself may continue. And the individual no longer is in an untenable disequilibrium.

Another component of a medical crisis relates to the flux of defense mechanisms. The failure of immature, neurotic, and mature defenses (Meissner, Mack, & Semrad, 1975) in the context of the psychosocial medical crisis throws the individual back to primitive narcissistic ego-defense mechanisms. During an interpersonal crisis narcissistic ego defenses of projection, distortion, and even denial may emerge. When the patient's narcissistic ego-defense mechanisms also fail to cope effectively at a turning point, then psychosis, flight, suicide, or even homicide may emerge as alternatives. Some patients or their families accuse, denigrate, manipulate, and even litigate (Lindeman, 1944).

Of course, not all patients in a medical crisis regress, accuse, or flee. Some engage with "personality," e.g., cheery comments coupled with compulsive giving of compliments or gifts. Some patients with interpersonal crises and with intrapersonal crises become depressed; others disengage (Weisman and Hackett, 1961). Finally, as in life outside the hospital, there are a few patients who grow during their crises. After all, dying is a phase of living, and living can be a growth experience—or its opposite, a disintegrating experience.

A third component to be considered in a medical crisis is the influence of the sick bed (Van den Berg, 1966). Illness at home is usually more comforting, but often care from the attending physician is problematic. In a hospital setting the physician will certainly observe and listen to the patient, but at times the physician will not have seen what the patient is up to nor have heard what is going on. The patient is then faced with the paradox of a nontherapeutic treatment setting. Illness itself produces regression. Additionally, the nontherapeutic nature of staff behaviors may augment it. Why does this occur? Medical and nursing staff, because of work stress, pressure of duties, or personal inclinations, often cope by becoming task-oriented or disease-oriented rather than person-oriented. Staff may isolate affect; use cliches, euphemisms, and rituals; and employ distracting techniques to avoid perceiving and feeling overwhelmed. Clearly, a better understanding of crises and how to deal with them would benefit medical and nursing staff care.

THERAPEUTIC INTERVENTIONS

To help our patients grow at their turning points or to let them grow without our interference is a real challenge. Typically, these patients need rest, shelter, protection, and support. The therapist provides interest, kindness, and professional competence. His/her presence provides the possibility of renewed hope (Straker, 1975). As Finkel (1982) puts it, "When in crisis, a patient can be viewed operationally as a child temporarily in need of a parent." Hence, the therapist may provide structure, give advice, make judgmental statements, provide alternative solutions, support dependency needs, relieve guilt, and manipulate the environment and support system in useful ways. But Nell's physician, by using so-called benign neglect, frustrated her planning a well-thought-out way of dealing with her impersonal and intrapersonal crisis. The evolving disintegration of her ALS and the shattering of her self-esteem precipitated an interpersonal crisis. Norman's CCU staff used professional reassurance to indicate that no slight was intended. Unfortunately, they did not perceive that his longstanding, profound lack of self-esteem necessitated their taking an extra step: he needed to be treated in a special fashion in a potential "against medical advice" situation. Both patients needed extra *understanding* and *involvement* although not necessarily extra *time* to help them negotiate a crucial developmental phase. Marie with her ovarian carcinoma and Mandy with her leukemia had that extra understanding and involvement, to the actual delight of the hospital staff. A successful network formed around them. Staff satisfaction in dealing with Marie's and Mandy's crises would certainly be rated as higher than that for Nell's and Norman's.

Are there any differentiating principles in dealing with an intrapersonal medical crisis and an interpersonal medical crisis? Since the individual with an intrapersonal crisis sees frustrations of the achievement of goals as coming from within, the therapeutic task is to support the individual in achieving his/her goal(s) or some approximation of the goal(s). If the patient asks for a lethal pill, one supports the patient's wish for a good death or pain relief, since presumably we can't initiate euthanasia. If the patient chooses to withdraw, one can support this, but it may be appropriate to see if there might be some other goal that would be even more acceptable though not dreamed of—honor, respect, dignity. The consultant helps the patient to achieve the patient's goal at the turning point.

An interpersonal medical crisis demands a different therapeutic approach. One can help the individual to reassess the situation and resolve the crisis by a change in perception; one can intervene with a significant other—or one can actually become a significant other. Here the locus of the problem is seen as outside the patient. The patient's anguish is that he/she is powerless to resolve the crisis. The consultant's role is to defuse the situation, reestablish the status quo, and/or work with, banish, or "shape up" the significant other (administrator, physician, family member, priest) whose actions or inactions have initiated the crisis.

CRISIS INTERVENTION AND CONSULTATION/LIAISON PSYCHIATRY

How does the role of the crisis intervener fit with the usually established job description for the consultation liaison (C/L) psychiatrist? Typically, the C/L psychiatrist cares for the delirious, demented, and depressed, the paranoid, petulant, perturbed, and perturbing. C/L psychiatrists also resolve patient/ staff and staff/staff conflicts. But rarely in the typical activities of C/L psychiatry does the word *crisis* appear (Hackett, 1976; Hackett & Cassem, 1978; Karasu, Plutchik, Conte, Siegel, & Steinmuller, 1977).

Why? I think we tend to take crisis work for granted; so accustomed are we to the very nature of our work that almost every time we are consulted a turning point has been reached, and the outcome often hangs precariously in the balance. Will the patient sue, sign out against advice, pull out the IV, refuse surgery, or continue to "tongue" the medication? Will the family continue to hound the nursing staff to the point that care for other patients on the unit will be compromised?

C/L psychiatrists have traditionally tended to see the real benefit of their work as promoting growth in patients and in staff, an activity that gets to the heart of why many psychiatrists went into their specialty. Curiously, though, C/L psychiatrists often do not see their primary role as crisis interveners, nor have they tended to sell this role to third-party payers or hospital administrators.

Let me make an analogy. If you ask a surgeon what he/she does, he/she may say, "Abdominal surgery, gallbladders, hernias, cancer." Right away we understand. It would be most unlikely that the surgeon would respond to your questions by describing his/her activities as "cutting through the skin, arteries, and veins and then tying off vessels." In a similar fashion almost everyone we see in consultation liaison work is in some sort of crisis. That crisis, if left unattended, can be measured in inappropriately spent monies and unnecessarily experienced anguish. But typically, we say that we resolve patient conflicts, patient-staff conflicts, staff-staff conflicts, treat psychiatric disease, and promote psychological growth. And then inevitably, administrators and third-party payers don't have a clear idea of what we do for the patient or the hospital! Perhaps it is time that C/L psychiatrists change the name of the game to *crisis management work* and the name of their teams to *crisis management teams,* so that third-party payers can understand C/L activities and fund them appropriately (Fenton & Guggenheim, 1981; Hales & Fink, 1982).

Crises often occur throughout a medical service. At times they are not perceived because of hurry with the rush of affairs, temporary psychological closure, social decorum, or genuine imperception of psychosocial events. Likewise, change occurs frequently in medical settings, medical staff often become desensitized to relevant, important psychosocial complications. What *doesn't* change is that turning points, points of no return, occur daily in the lives of our patients whether or not we are there to help out.

REFERENCES

Fenton, B. J., & Guggenheim, F. G. (1981). Consultation-liaison psychiatry and funding: Why can't Alice find Wonderland? *General Hospital Psychiatry, 3,* 255–260.

Festinger, L. (1957). *A theory of cognitive dissonance.* New York: Harper + Row.

Finkel, I. B., Kornfeld, D. S., & Finkel, J. B. (Eds.), (1982). Psychotherapy in medical practice. *Psychiatric management for medical practitioners.* (pp. 47–60) New York: Grune & Stratton.

France, K. (1982). *Crisis intervention: A handbook of immediate person-to-person help.* Springfield, IL: Charles C. Thomas.

Guggenheim, F. G. (1978). A marketplace model of consultation psychiatry in the general hospital. *American Journal of Psychiatry, 135,* 1380–1383.

Hackett, T. P. (1976). The psychiatrist's view of the ICU: Vital signs stable but outlook guarded. *Psychiatric Annals, 6,* 14–27.

Hackett, T. P., & Cassem, N. H. (1978). *Massachusetts General Hospital handbook of general hospital psychiatry.* St. Louis: C. V. Mosby Company.

Hales, R. E., & Fink, P. J. (1982). A modest proposal for consultation-liaison psychiatry in the 1980s. *American Journal of Psychiatry, 139,* 1015–1021.

Karasu, T. B., Plutchik, R., Conte, H., Siegel, B., Steinmuller, R., & Rosenbaum, M. (1977). What do physicians want from a psychiatric consultation service? *Comprehensive Psychiatry, 18,* 73–81.

Leo, J. (1980). How to commit suicide. *Time,* July 7, 1980, p. 49.

Lindemann, E. (1944). Symptomatology and management of acute grief. *American Journal of Psychiatry, 101,* 141–148.

Meissner, W., Mack, J., & Semrad, E. (1975). Classical psychoanalysis. In A. Freedman, H. Kaplan, & B. Dadock (Eds.), *Comprehensive textbook of psychiatry II.* (pp. 534–536) Baltimore: Williams and Wilkins.

Puryear, D. (1979). *Helping people in crisis.* San Francisco: Jossey-Bass.

Satir, V. (1972). *Peoplemaking*. Palo Alto, CA: Science and Behavior Books.

Schwab, J. J. (1968). *Handbook of psychiatric consultation*. New York: Appleton-Century-Crofts.

Straker, M. (1975). The psychiatric emergency. In R. O. Pasnau (Ed.), *Consultation-liaison psychiatry*. (p. 190) New York: Grune & Stratton.

Van den Berg, J. H. (1966). *The psychology of the sickbed*. Pittsburgh: Duquesne University Press.

Weisman, A. D., & Hackett, T. P. (1961). Predilection to death: Death and dying as a psychiatric problem. *Psychosomatic Medicine, 13,* 232–256.

Chapter 2

ORGANIC BRAIN SYNDROMES

Robert Roessler and Gregory Graham

Organic brain syndromes (OBS) are frequent in patients who are physically ill. They signal the presence of significant organic disease that may or may not have been diagnosed. Whereas severe OBS is usually recognized, lesser degrees may not be. When patients suffer from OBS, they are emotionally distressed, and they behave in ways that endanger them and that obstruct effective treatment. This chapter focuses primarily on recognizing the symptoms and signs of lesser degrees of OBS, because they are more likely to be unrecognized. It also discusses their etiology and their symptomatic and etiologic treatment. It is addressed to primary physicians who are the first to see patients during their hospital stay.

Although there are few well-designed studies of the prevalence of OBS among patients in general hospitals, it is substantial. Delirium and dementia, the most common OBS, are the principal subjects of this chapter. Lipowski (1980) has estimated that delirium is present in 5 to 15 percent of all patients on general medical and surgical wards and in 2 to 30 percent of patients in intensive care units. Dementia has been estimated at somewhat less than 1 percent in the general population (Butler, 1978). However, because dementia occurs primarily in the elderly, and the elderly are more likely to be hospitalized, the prevalence among hospital patients is considerably greater (Blessed & Wilson, 1982). Consultation/liaison (C/L) psychiatrists typically report that 10 to 20 percent of the patients they are asked to see are suffering from OBS. They also report that 20 to 30 percent of these syndromes have not been recognized by the physicians requesting consultation (Denny, Quass, & Rich, 1966; Shevitz, Silverfarb, & Lipowski, 1976). Whatever the exact frequency of OBS in all general hospitals, it is high, particularly in tertiary-care hospitals.

Not only is the frequency high but it is becoming higher. The increase is related in part to the increase in the number and proportion of the elderly in the population. The elderly are at great risk for primary degenerative dementia (senile dementia of the Alzheimer type [SDAT]), the risk increasing with each decade of life (Hendrix, 1978). Because the "older old" are increasing most rapidly, one writer has predicted "a deluge of dementia," primarily because of SDAT (Wells, 1981). The elderly are also at greater risk for the development of delirium (Lipowski, 1983). This risk is related partly to dementia, which increases the risk for delirium. Among patients over sixty years who were admitted to a psychiatric ward, 50 percent were diagnosed as having "acute brain syndrome" (delirium), and 80 percent of those with delirium also were diagnosed as having "chronic brain syndrome" (dementia) (Bedford, 1959).

The risk for delirium in the elderly also is related to the prevalence of chronic diseases among older persons. Many of these diseases—coronary and myocardial disease, congestive heart failure, diabetes, cancer, renal failure, malnutrition and dehydration, cerebrovascular disease, and sensory impairments (blindness and deafness)—carry an increased risk for delirium. Because of their greater incidence of chronic disease the elderly are also more likely to be taking medications that, separately or in combination, may produce delirium (Vestal, 1978). They are especially likely to be taking psychotropic drugs, many of which have anticholinergic effects (Hall, Feinsilver, & Holt, 1981; C.E. Sermas, *this volume*). Because of the many chronic illnesses, such as arthritis, that are associated with pain they also use analgesics and anti-inflammatory medications more frequently. Psychotropics, analgesics, and anti-inflammatory drugs all carry a significant risk of delirium. Additional medications that commonly precipitate delirium in the elderly are sedative hypnotics, digitalis, and diuretics. Not only are older patients more likely to be taking drugs but their metabolism of drugs is more likely to be impaired; the risk of delirium is therefore increased further (Lipowski, 1980; C.E. Sermas, *this volume*).

The elderly are also more likely to undergo surgery, and the incidence of postoperative delirium among them is high (Millar, 1981). Because of sensory impairments and infirmities they are also at greater risk for accidents. Some of these accidents involve head trauma, which may produce delirium. Many others involve subsequent immobilization, infection, dehydration, and related electrolyte imbalances, all of which increase the risk for delirium. Clearly, the possibility of delirium and dementia in all older patients must always be given high priority in differential diagnosis.

Although the elderly are more likely to suffer from dementia and delirium, younger patients are also at risk. Young adults are more likely to be involved in vehicular accidents than are older adults and therefore to sustain head injuries (Levin & Grossman, 1978). They are also more likely to abuse substances, including alcohol, cannabis, phencyclidine, hallucinogens, barbiturates and other hypnotics, amphetamine and other sympathomimetics, opioids and other analgesics, and cocaine (Fishburne, Abelson, & Crisin, 1980). These substances, and withdrawal from their chronic use, are associated with a very high risk of delirium. Their abuse also is related to a higher risk of vehicular accidents, which are in turn related to risk of delirium and dementia. Nor are younger persons immune from many of the diseases that afflict the elderly; they too may suffer congestive heart failure, infections, renal failure, cancer, diabetes, and dietary deficiencies. When they do, they are at lesser but still appreciable risk for delirium.

RECOGNITION OF DEMENTIA AND DELIRIUM

Recognizing the patient with dementia and/or delirium may pose no problem if it is severe, although the clinical picture is sometimes confused with "functional" psychosis (psychosis presumed to be based in psychological conflict without central nervous system pathology). However, a significant proportion of patients suffering mild to moderate dementia and delirium go unrecognized, as we noted earlier. When they remain unrecognized, the consequences may be crucial to the patient's welfare.

One serious consequence may be the failure to diagnose the presence of potentially fatal and treatable disease. In older patients particularly, but in younger ones as well, a mild to moderate degree of delirium may be the only immediate evidence of serious pathology. If the delirium is overlooked, the underlying pathology often also will be unrecognized and the patient therefore not treated. Undiagnosed disease is probably at least partly responsible for the high mortality reported among delirious patients. Weddington (1982) and Rabins and Folstein (1982) reported that about one-third of delirious patients died within 3 months, for example. Guze and Cantrell (1964) reported that higher mortality occurred in younger delirious patients as well as in older patients.

Another common consequence of not recognizing delirium and dementia is the failure of the patient to comply with treatment: failing to take essential medication or taking too much; engaging in proscribed activities or failing to engage in prescribed activities; and failing to adhere to dietary restrictions. Still another consequence of the failure to recognize OBS is accidental injury, particularly at night. The patient may become so disoriented, delusional, and agitated that he injures himself. The patient also may injure others, although this is rare. Finally, but also important because dementia and delirium are usually associated with considerable subjective distress, the patient may suffer unnecessarily.

In summary, the possibility of OBS always must be considered in any patient with a physical illness. It is especially important to consider in patients who are older, injured, febrile, post-surgical, acutely or chronically ill, or receiving multiple medications. Combinations of two or more of these make the probability of impaired cerebral function even greater. When the possibility of OBS is considered, what is the evidence indicating its presence?

The diagnostic classification currently used by most psychiatrists is that described in the third edition of the *Diagnostic and Statistical Manual of Mental Disorders* (DSM-III) (1980). DSM-III differentiates between OBS and *organic mental disorders.* OBS are defined as constellations of behavioral signs and symptoms without reference to etiology, whereas organic mental disorders designate an organic syndrome in which the specific etiology is known or presumed. OBS are subdivided into delirium and dementia, in both of which cognitive impairment is relatively great; and further, into amnestic, organic hallucinosis, organic delusional, organic affective, and organic personality syndromes, in which the named symptoms predominate and other cognitive impairment is relatively limited.

DSM-III defines delirium as a syndrome of central nervous system dysfunctions characterized by varying degrees of impairment in attention, perception, orientation, memory, and thinking. Affective and autonomic lability and abnormal movements are frequent in severe delirium. Onset is usually rapid over hours or days. The level of consciousness in delirious patients fluctuates. The fluctuations typically occur over the course of hours. Level of consciousness may range from semicomatose to hypervigilant. These changes are often out of phase with the usual diurnal sleep pattern and accompany other impairments in mental functioning. The impairments, particularly those in attention, are frequently worse at night ("sundowning"). Related to the changes in the level of consciousness there are also impairments in attention.

Delirious patients have difficulty in focusing, shifting, and sustaining attention (Lipowski, 1980). In part because of these deficits they have difficulty in comprehending questions and instructions and may misperceive both the meaning of words and discrete environmental and internal stimuli. Illusions and hallucinations are common, particularly in severe delirium, and are more common when sensory input is reduced (at night, for example). Both illusions and hallucinations are more commonly visual but may occur in any sensory modality.

Disorientation is always present in delirium but may fluctuate, the degree ranging from mild misidentification of time of day or day of week to severe (misidentification of year). Place identification is often impaired, varying in degree from mis-naming of hospital to severe (at home). Orientation for person usually remains intact in milder degrees of delirium but may be absent in more severe degrees. In severe delirium orientation may not be testable. Memory (if testable) is always impaired, varying with the severity of delirium. Recent memory is always affected, and intermediate and long-term memory is impaired in more severe delirium. Speech, reflecting the underlying dis-order of thinking, is usually slowed and fragmented, the pa-tient losing the goal of thought. Perseveration of speech and repetitive motor behavior may be present. The capacity to ab-stract is impaired and is reflected in an inability to define sim-ilarities and dissimilarities, for example.

Emotional symptoms are common, including anxiety, irri-tability, anger, depression, euphoria, and apathy. Fear is often present, particularly if the patient experiences illusions or hal-lucinations. Emotions are often labile, with sudden and unpre-dictable onset. Crying, moaning, cursing, and muttering are common, especially at night.

Psychomotor activity is typically variable, ranging from restlessness and hyperactivity to apathy and sluggishness. Patho-logical neurological signs are uncommon except for abnormal movements including tremor, multifocal myoclonus (asymmet-ric, nonrhythmic contractions of muscles or muscle groups at rest), and asterixis ("flapping tremor").

Autonomic nervous system changes may be present, espe-cially if the delirium is due to substance intoxication or with-drawal. Symptoms include pupillary dilation, elevated pulse and blood pressure, tachycardia, fever, perspiration, nausea and vomiting.

The *essential DSM-III criteria for a diagnosis of delirium* are reduced awareness of the environment with reduced capacity to shift, focus, and sustain attention; disorientation and memory impairment; relatively sudden onset (usually hours or days) and fluctuation over a day; evidence of an organic etiology for brain dysfunction; and at least two of the following: perceptual dis-turbance, intermittently incoherent speech, insomnia or day-time drowsiness, increased or decreased psychomotor activity.

The *essential DSM-III criteria for the diagnosis of dementia* are a loss of intellectual abilities of sufficient severity to interfere with social or occupational functioning; memory impairment; level of consciousness not clouded; at least one of the following: impaired abstraction, impaired judgment, other disturbances of higher cortical function (aphasia, apraxia, agnosia, constructional difficulty), personality change; and one of the following: a defined etiologic factor or a presumption of such a factor, if "the behavioral change represents cognitive impairment in a number of areas."

Substance-Induced Organic Mental Disorders

The DSM-III classification of organic mental disorders includes primary degenerative dementia of presenile and senile onset, multi-infarct dementia, and a number of substance-induced intoxications and withdrawal syndromes. The latter include alcohol; barbiturates and other sedatives or hypnotics; opioids; cocaine; amphetamines and other sympathomimetics; phencyclidine (PCP) and similarly acting arylcyclohexylamines; hallucinogens such as LSD, dimethyltriptamine and other substances chemically related to catecholamines; cannabis; tobacco; and caffeine. Certain of these etiologic classifications are subdivided. Dementias are qualified as "with delirium," "with delusions," "with depression," and "uncomplicated." Diagnoses in the alcohol-induced group of disorders include intoxication, withdrawal, withdrawal hallucinosis, amnestic disorder, and dementia.

Certain of the etiologic agents in the substance-abuse organic mental disorders have relatively distinctive clinical features related to their pharmacologic properties or to specific physiologic effects of their withdrawal. Lacrimation and rhinorrhea, pupillary dilation, piloerection, yawning, and fever are common in patients suffering from opioid withdrawal, for example. This contrasts to the pupillary constriction associated with opioid intoxication and with the nystagmus, ataxia, and dysarthria more characteristic of PCP and alcohol intoxication. Such differences can assist the physician seeing the patient for the first time in identifying specific etiologic substances or classes of substances and are helpful in choosing specific treatment, such as naloxone for opioid withdrawal.

However, the various substance-abuse organic mental disorders are more similar than dissimilar in the signs and symptoms that are observable by the physician on initial contact. Evidence of autonomic hyperactivity (tachycardia, sweating, elevated blood pressure), affective disturbances (anxiety, irritability, apathy, euphoria, depression), hallucinations, delusions, and psychomotor hypo- and hyperactivity, and most important, disturbances in attention, memory, orientation, perception, and thinking are common to many substance-intoxication and withdrawal syndromes. Moreover, from the standpoint of the physician who is seeing the patient for the first time, an essential criterion for each specific substance-induced diagnosis is evidence of ingestion of a specific substance. Such historical evidence is often lacking, at least initially, because the delirious and/or demented patient's history is unreliable because of memory impairment. Reliable alternative sources of such information are also frequently not immediately available. Similarly, laboratory evidence of the presence of toxins or of metabolic disorder are usually lacking initially.

THE WORKUP

There is much overlap in the criteria for delirium and dementia. For the physician initially evaluating a patient with OBS, distinguishing between the two may be very difficult. Both can involve changes in sensorium, affect, memory, cognition, and orientation. Furthermore, delirium frequently complicates dementia, resulting in a mixed clinical picture. Of critical help in differential diagnosis at the time of initial evaluation is the length of history of the impairment. In delirium the onset is relatively acute. In dementia the onset is usually insidious. This history, combined with the characteristics of dementia and delirium described above, gives some good indications as to which syndrome is present. Nonetheless, in many cases, particularly in the absence of adequate history, a precise diagnosis is not possible. In all cases, however, an extensive workup is indicated to determine a specific organic etiology.

The workup is organized operationally from the first patient contact through later identification of specific etiologies and specific treatment. These operations are organized in relation to the following sequential questions: (1) Is he/she a member of a high-risk group? (2) If so, is there evidence in the patient's behavior during the examination and interview that suggests possible delirium and/or dementia? (3) If there is, what are the results of a formal mental status examination? (4) If there is evidence of OBS on the mental status examination, what treatment should be instituted immediately? (5) What further information should be sought to identify the probable specific cause(s) of the OBS? (6) If probable cause(s) are identified, what steps can be taken to increase the accuracy of identification? (7) What treatment should be instituted to ameliorate the specific cause(s)? We will illustrate this operational strategy through a case history, following the patient throughout her hospital course from admission to discharge.

Risk Factors

The patient was a sixty-five-year-old widow, a retired executive who was admitted to the hospital following an automobile accident. She was brought to the hospital by a city ambulance, and details of the accident were not immediately available. She had sustained multiple lacerations with significant blood loss and a compound fracture of her left tibia. It was not clear whether she had sustained a head injury. She was semiconscious and unable to give any history. Routine laboratory data was within normal limits except for the evidence of blood loss. Under general anesthesia the lacerations were sutured, and an open reduction of the fracture was accomplished. She received 2 units of whole blood. She regained consciousness after 2 h in the recovery room and was moved to a private room. Postoperatively, promethazine hydrochloride, 50 mg, and meperidine hydrochloride, 50 mg, q4h, p.r.n., were prescribed intramuscularly for the control of pain.

The patient's daughter informed the surgeon the day after

admission that the patient had suffered from rheumatoid arthritis for about 15 years and had been using ibuprofen, 400 mg, every 6 h for the relief of pain for an unknown period. She also had a history of duodenal ulcer and had recently been taking cimetidine, 400 mg, at bedtime for about 3 months. Following her retirement 6 months previously, there was a question of whether she had become depressed. She was taking amitriptyline hydrochloride, 25 mg, t.i.d., and 75 mg at bedtime. The surgeon therefore prescribed the ibuprofen, cimetidine, and amitriptyline in the previously prescribed doses.

This patient was at risk for OBS for several reasons. She was sixty-five years old and therefore at risk for dementia. She suffered from two known chronic illnesses, arthritis and duodenal ulcer. She was taking five drugs that can produce delirium: ibuprofen and cimetidine for arthritis and duodenal ulcer, amitriptyline for depression (at a dose high for her age), and promethazine and meperidine for pain. She had experienced severe trauma and associated blood loss and had undergone general anesthesia and extensive surgery, all associated with increased risk for delirium. Because of the multiple drugs she was taking she was also at risk for drug interactions with drugs used during and after surgery (C.E. Sermas, *this volume*). Depression preoperatively increases risk for delirium postoperatively. The risk factors present in this patient not only point to the likelihood of OBS but also point to possible causes.

Multiple risk factors in hospitalized patients are common. This is particularly true of older patients with a history of chronic illness and associated polypharmacy. Multiple risk factors in younger patients are less common but still frequent and include chronic illness, multiple drugs (prescribed and nonprescribed), drug interactions, alcohol, and trauma.

Examination and Interview

Forty-eight hours after surgery a psychiatric consultation was requested by the patient's surgeon because of the patient's questionable history of depression and because he felt that she appeared depressed. Before interviewing the patient, the psychiatrist reviewed her chart. She noted the risk factors for OBS and also read in the nurses' notes for the previous night that the patient had slept poorly and during one check had apparently been very frightened, apparently mistaking the nurse's flashlight for the headlights of an oncoming car. She was quickly reassured when reminded she was in the hospital following an accident. The psychiatrist also noted that the patient's pulse rate was 100, temperature was normal, and blood pressure was 160/95. The patient had been receiving all medications as prescribed, including the p.r.n. analgesics q4h.

When the psychiatrist introduced herself, the patient seemed somewhat surprised. The psychiatrist was surprised in turn, because the surgeon had said that the patient had agreed to the consultation. The psychiatrist explained the reason for the consultation, and the patient agreed to it. The psychiatrist observed that the patient appeared about her stated age, was somewhat disheveled, and looked flushed. She denied chest pain. Her facial expression was strained and anxious and she was often restless, rearranging the bedclothing frequently. The psychiatrist also observed that the patient was distracted by sounds from the hall and had difficulty in sustaining her attention to questions, often returning to her concern that her daughter was late for a visit. She also noted that the patient's responses to questions were delayed at times and that she spoke slowly, sometimes losing the goal of her thoughts. The patient said that she had been "at loose ends" following her retirement but denied vegetative symptoms and denied that she felt depressed currently. She confirmed the history of arthritis and ulcer and reported additional details. She knew why she was in the hospital but could not recall the events leading up to the accident or the events following it. She thought she had been in the hospital "about a week." When her memory failed her, she became distressed and anxious. With reassurance and a change of topic her distress was quickly relieved. On two occasions, when speaking of apparently innocuous subjects, she suddenly cried but just as suddenly stopped. When describing certain events that had occurred prior to her accident, she had difficulty in recalling dates even approximately. She had been living alone, she said, partly because her only daughter lived in another city but primarily because "I've always wanted to be independent." Her memory for remote events was intact, and she spoke in great detail about her business career, with obvious pride in her ability to manage successfully the sometimes competing demands of motherhood and those of her career.

At this point there was additional evidence that increased the probability that the patient was suffering from an OBS. The patient had slept poorly and had experienced a nighttime illusion of a nature that suggested simultaneous disorientation. This, in combination with the absence of any obvious daytime disorientation, might have been evidence of a fluctuating level of consciousness that was worse at night; this is characteristic of delirium but also occurs in demented patients. There was also an elevated pulse rate and blood pressure, flushed facies, and excessive perspiration, suggestive of autonomic hyperactivity. These need to be evaluated against a baseline, of course, and such information was lacking. They also must be evaluated in relation to other possible causes of autonomic hyperactivity, such as infection, myocardial infarction, pulmonary embolus, or internal bleeding. There was also evidence during the interview that the patient had difficulty in sustaining her attention, was distractable, showed increased and decreased psychomotor activity, had impaired recent memory, and was slightly disoriented. Note that there was also some evidence of the personality of the patient—"independent."

Similar information from conversation with patients and from observation of them is available to all professionals. If they are alerted by the presence of risk factors for OBS, they will be alerted also to these relatively subtle changes in behavior that if present are additional indications of the presence of OBS. Tentative evidence of OBS in the interview should never be dismissed as fatigue or preoccupation; formal testing (mental status examination) will reveal more definitive evidence of presence or absence of OBS.

Mental Status Examination

After completing the initial history the psychiatrist told the patient that she needed to ask some additional questions. Some of these, she said, might seem strange but they were important. She then asked the patient her full name, address, and telephone number, which the patient readily supplied. (It agreed with data the daughter supplied for the chart.) She then asked the time of day, day of the week, month, and year. The patient said it was Friday (actually Monday), that it was afternoon (correct after looking at her watch and out the window), that it was August (correct), and that it was 1983 (correct). Asked for the name of the hospital, the patient said, "I know; I just can't think of it." She knew the city. The psychiatrist asked the patient what she had had for lunch (after checking earlier on the actual lunch); the patient could not remember and was distressed but then dismissed it—"Oh, that's not important."

The psychiatrist then asked the patient to identify three objects and to remember them until asked later. Later she could remember only one. She could repeat five digits forward but only two backward. Again she was distressed but was immediately relieved by gentle reassurance. Asked to subtract serial sevens from 100 in her head, she had no difficulty reaching 93, but each successive subtraction of seven was progressively slower, with increasing errors. Again the patient was distressed and said, "I did that in my work often, and it was easy then." When told she would probably be able to do so again when she was better, she was again quickly reassured. Abstraction was tested by asking the patient to say how an apple and pear were alike; she said they were both fruit. When asked how they were different she said, "That's silly; they're not." When asked to interpret the meaning of proverbs, all of her answers were concrete; for example, when asked the meaning of "People who live in glass houses should not throw stones," she said, "The glass would break." Asked to read aloud a passage from a book, she quickly dismissed it after several errors with "That just doesn't make sense." When encouraged to try again, she refused with great irritation: "I don't see what any of this has to do with the reason I'm here."

At this point the psychiatrist returned to the patient's earlier life. When the patient had difficulty in remembering the medications she had taken and their frequency, the psychiatrist asked for permission to talk with her daughter to get that and other information. The patient agreed: "She can tell you some

of those things better than I. I'm tired." The psychiatrist then
said she could certainly understand that it was difficult to answer so many questions when she was ill and had trouble thinking and keeping track of what was happening. The patient
looked relieved and said, "Yes, I'm not usually like this. Do you
think that will improve?" The psychiatrist replied that she
thought it would. She then left, saying she would return later.

After the formal mental status examination there was definite evidence of an OBS of mild to moderate degree: disorientation to time, impaired recent memory, impaired retention,
difficulty with serial subtraction, "organic affectivity" (sudden
onset without appropriate stimulus), impaired abstraction and
concrete thinking, and rationalization and denial of the importance of these. It was not clear whether the OBS was a delirium
or dementia or both. The DSM-III criteria for dementia were
met. However, all of the foregoing may be present in delirium
as well, as we noted earlier. There was no definitive information on the nature of the onset of these symptoms at this junc-
ture; they might have been present before the accident or may
have begun after the accident. The crucial information *was*
available, however; the patient was suffering from an OBS.
Whether it is dementia or delirium, a reversible cause must be
sought. Further information from the daughter might provide
a basis for identifying the cause. In the meantime, however,
symptomatic treatment should begin immediately and steps be
taken to reduce the effect of suspected causes.

Immediate Treatment and Further Information

The psychiatrist called the surgeon and reported that there
was definite evidence of an OBS. She told him that there were
a number of possible causes and enumerated them. She said that
the ibuprofen, cimetidine, and amitriptyline could be acting
separately or together to produce the OBS. She suggested that
a rheumatologist and gastroenterologist be asked to consult on
the current need for the first two drugs and recommended that
the amitriptyline dose be reduced gradually. The surgeon
agreed. She also suggested that the promethazine and meperidine be reduced as soon as possible, and the surgeon agreed,

adding that the patient's pain had already diminished considerably. The surgeon also asked that the psychiatrist write orders for any diagnostic tests that she felt might assist in clarifying the cause(s) and that she write the order for reducing the amitriptyline. The psychiatrist said that she would speak with the patient's daughter regarding the patient's mental condition prior to the accident and also advise her that private duty nurses would be desirable if that was financially feasible. The surgeon thanked the psychiatrist, who said that she would be in touch again when more information was available.

The psychiatrist then spoke with the patient's daughter, who had arrived to visit the patient in the meantime. The psychiatrist described the current situation to the daughter and the possible reasons for the OBS and the decision to reduce and discontinue the medications as soon as possible. The daughter said that she had had little recent contact with her mother because she lived in another city, but she said that she had not noticed any memory problems or difficulty in her mother's thinking in the contacts she had had by telephone in the month prior to the accident. She gave the psychiatrist the name and telephone number of her mother's neighbor and friend who had seen her almost daily prior to the accident. She also said that neither she nor her mother could afford private-duty nurses around the clock. The psychiatrist suggested a night nurse, explaining that this was likely to be the most difficult period for the patient; the daughter agreed. The psychiatrist suggested a television set, a semiprivate room with another patient, and a bed next to a window to increase sensory input during the day when she did not have visitors.

They then talked more about the patient and her history. The daughter said that the patient was the oldest of four children and had become a second mother to her younger siblings because her mother had suffered from periodic cardiac decompensation. Her mother had died when the patient was twelve. After the mother's death the patient had assumed full responsibility for the care of the home and her younger siblings. Her father provided adequate financial support but little help in the home. The patient left home to go to college at seventeen and thereafter returned infrequently, partly because she married at age nineteen while still a student. After college the patient supported her husband and herself by working as a secretary while he worked on an advanced degree. After her husband completed his degree and took a teaching job, the patient remained at home. The daughter was born when the patient was twenty-five; there were no other children. Five years later the patient's husband died in an accident, and the patient returned to work as a secretary. She advanced rapidly to an executive level but managed to spend considerable time with the daughter. When she could not, she would explain and apologize profusely to the daughter. The patient had a few short-term relationships with men but never thought seriously of remarrying. She continued to be promoted, and after her daughter left for college, she devoted herself almost exclusively to work. Occasionally, she took brief vacations but was always restless during them and anxious to return to work.

The daughter said that her mother had suffered intermittently from ulcer symptoms "for as long as I can remember." The patient's rheumatoid arthritis had begun when the patient was in her mid-forties but had rarely been incapacitating; when she had a flare-up of symptoms "she would grin and bear it." The daughter was uncertain how long she had taken ibuprofen but thought it was "several months." Immediately following her retirement the patient seemed depressed but had no early morning awakening or weight loss. The daughter had asked her to move to her home, but the patient had always refused, sometimes adding she didn't want to be a burden. To the daughter's knowledge, the patient had never been depressed prior to her retirement. She thought she might have been depressed following her husband's death because of remarks her grandfather had made about her mother's behavior during that period.

Following this conversation the psychiatrist wrote a consultation note on the patient's chart and wrote orders for an EEG, ECG, computed tomography (CT) of the brain, B_{12} and folate determinations, and repeat hematocrit, electrolytes, and blood gases. She also wrote an order for the gradual reduction of the amitriptyline.

She then spoke with the patient's primary nurse and informed her of the OBS and the possible causes. She suggested that the nurse post a sign in large letters, reminding the patient to call if she needed anything, but also to check the patient frequently for needs nevertheless, because of the patient's fierce independence. At the same time she should allow the patient to do anything she could do for herself without risking injury. She asked the nurse to speak slowly, clearly, and somewhat louder than usual in order to obtain and maintain the patient's attention; to remind her frequently of where she was and why because of the patient's memory impairment; and to reassure and distract her when she was distressed. The psychiatrist also asked her to ask the daughter to bring familiar photographs and other personal belongings to the patient's room. She also asked her to inform the night nurse of the nursing procedures and to ask the night nurse to leave a night-light on for the patient so that she could orient herself quickly if she awoke during the night. The primary nurse agreed, adding that the patient was "a model patient, but she does try to do too much for herself."

The psychiatrist then called the patient's neighbor. The neighbor reported that she had seen the patient daily but had not noted any change in the patient's memory or thinking prior to the accident. She had noted these difficulties when visiting the patient in the hospital. She confirmed that the patient was "a very independent person—she could be dying and never ask for help."

Having established the presence of an OBS, the psychiatrist immediately initiated symptomatic treatment and began the search for further data to clarify the cause. She also took some initial steps to reduce the effects of some of the likely causes.

The reasons for the various treatment decisions are directly related to the nature of the sensory, behavioral, and emotional aspects of the pathology characteristic of OBS and to the personality of the patient. Except for those related to personality, these treatment decisions are common to all patients suffering from OBS. They include minimizing the effects of the impairment of recent memory; augmenting sensory input and increasing its clarity, constancy, and familiarity; and reducing emotional distress. The latter include using the distractability characteristic of OBS to refocus the patient's attention away from the distressing topic. It did not include any medication.

Had the patient's subjective distress, behavioral disturbance, and insomnia been greater, haloperidol in small doses would have been useful. In older patients who are acutely ill, initial doses of 0.5 to 2.0 mg, t.i.d., with a p.r.n. nighttime dose, is often sufficient. If it is not, the dose may be titrated upward to the minimum effective dose. (It is advisable to consult a psychiatrist regarding an optimal dose and schedule of haloperidol because of the risks associated with overdose.) Although benzodiazepines or barbiturates were used in the past in these circumstances, in our experience they are more likely than haloperidol to increase the impairment of consciousness and also risk increasing the behavioral disturbance. This is particularly likely in older patients. Benzodiazepines and barbiturates should therefore be avoided. Physical restraint should be avoided; its use increases patients' fear and intensifies aggression. In an emergency it can be used briefly until haloperidol takes effect.

In this instance the psychiatrist now knew something about the "person who is the patient"—she was "very independent." Moreover, she was a person who had used her intellectual abilities with considerable success in her work, and there was suggestive evidence in her possible postretirement depression that her intellectual ability and interests were of great importance to her in maintaining her self-esteem. The psychiatrist therefore knew that the intellectual impairment associated with the OBS was likely to be very threatening to this patient. She therefore included the prescription that the patient be permitted to do everything that she could do for herself without risk of accidental injury. Loss of ability to interpret the environment correctly is threatening to every patient. Physicians and other professionals should indicate clearly to the patient that they recognize the presence of that problem and reassure the patient that it is temporary. Like every statement to the OBS patient, it must be repeated frequently because of the impairment of memory.

The psychiatrist spoke with the patient's daughter and with a neighbor. The information obtained from them not only provided a more complete picture of the patient as a person but also strongly suggested that the OBS did not precede the accident. Relatives and friends of OBS patients should always be consulted (with the patient's permission, if possible) to provide more reliable information than the patient can provide because of his/her impaired memory. These contacts also provide an opportunity to inform relatives and friends of the nature of the deficits and to suggest ways of relating to the patient that can reduce the patient's distress and behavioral disturbance.

The causes of OBS are innumerable. Any pathology that directly or indirectly influences cerebral physiology can produce it. General categories of organic pathology and pathophysiology associated with OBS are listed in Table 2-1.

The causes of OBS listed in Table 2-1 are not comprehensive but do provide a general framework for reviewing more specific ones. In terms of probability any evident pathology in any of the categories listed in Table 2-1 is a more probable cause. So are any drugs the patient is or has been taking. These include proprietary and over-the-counter medications and street drugs. Even drugs used in diagnostic procedures should be suspect; metrizamide, used in radiologic myelography, has been reported to produce OBS, for example (Penn & Mackenzie, 1983).

In the patient we have been discussing there was a history of trauma and surgery, rheumatoid arthritis, duodenal ulcer, and possible depression. All of these were associated with the use of medications. These pathologies and the medications associated with them are therefore the more likely causes. These should be pursued first because they are most likely to bring early remission and to contain diagnostic costs. The psychiatrist therefore took preliminary steps to reduce the medications and ordered an EEG, ECG, CT of the brain, B_{12} and folate, and repeat hematocrit, electrolytes, and blood gases. All of these were related to identifying more probable causes of the OBS in this patient. The EEG may support the presence of an OBS; if generalized slowing is present, it suggests the presence of cerebral dysfunction. (There is a caveat, however: a normal EEG does not rule out OBS.) The ECG was relevant to a possible cardiac basis for hypoxemia in a patient of this age. The CT of the brain was relevant to cerebral injury, although a normal CT does not rule out OBS. It also might be useful in ruling out less probable causes, such as neoplasm. B_{12} and folate are relevant to the

Table 2-1.   Categories of Organic Pathology and Pathophysiology Associated with Organic Brain Syndrome

I. Intracranial
   A. Trauma
      1. Open head wounds with direct cerebral damage
      2. Closed head injury with cerebral contusions (postconcussion syndrome), subdural, epidural, and subarachnoid hemorrhage
   B. Neoplasms, primary and metastatic
   C. Infections, including encephalitis, meningitis, and meningoencephalitis due to a variety of organisms
   D. Cerebrovascular disease, including cerebral arteriosclerosis, hemorrhage, thrombosis, multiple cerebral infarcts, and carotid stenosis
   E. Epilepsy and postictal states
   F. Degenerative disease, including senile dementia of the Alzheimer type, Parkinson's disease, Huntington's disease, and multiple sclerosis
   G. Normal-pressure hydrocephalus
II. Systemic
   A. Hypoxemia due to cardiac and/or pulmonary disease
   B. Drugs and drug interactions (intoxications and withdrawal)
      1. Psychotropics, particularly major tranquilizers and tricyclic antidepressants
      2. Analgesics, particularly opioids and synthetics
      3. Miscellaneous, including steroids, insulin, anticonvulsants, sympathomimetics, bromides, barbiturates, cardiac glycosides, alcohol, nonsteroid antiarthritics, cimetidine, and many others (see text)
   C. Endocrine (hyper- and hypofunction)
      1. Pituitary
      2. Pancreas
      3. Adrenal
      4. Thyroid
      5. Parathyroid
   D. Other organ malfunction
      1. Liver
      2. Kidney/bladder

3. Gastrointestinal, including constipation
4. Peripheral vascular disorders, including phlebitis
E. Electrolyte, fluid, and acid-base disturbances, particularly sodium, potassium, calcium, and magnesium changes; hypo- and hypervolemia; acidosis and alkalosis
F. Dietary deficiencies, including vitamin B_{12}, folate, and thiamine
G. Exogenous toxins, including heavy metals and carbon monoxide
H. Infections of any organ system

questionable history of depression in this patient and the possible dietary deficiency associated with it. The hematocrit is relevant to the history of injury and the possibility of continued blood loss and associated hypoxemia, as are the blood gases. The electrolytes in this patient might be disturbed for a variety of reasons but particularly because of the history of trauma and surgery. If all of the foregoing more likely causes were ruled out, then the search would turn toward identifying less probable causes.

Further Diagnostic Procedures

The following day the results of the above preliminary diagnostic work were available. The EEG showed generalized slowing, possibly supporting the presence of an OBS. The remaining tests were reported as within normal limits, ruling out any systemic cause of hypoxemia, electrolyte disturbance, and B_{12} or folate deficiency and making intracranial pathology less likely.

The psychiatrist then pursued the possibility of anticholinergic toxicity (Hall, Feinsilver, & Holt, 1981; Preskorn & Simpson, 1982). After explaining its purpose, she administered 1.0 mg of physostygmine intravenously slowly over 5 min and repeated portions of the mental status examination. The patient's mental status performance improved dramatically. After 15 min had passed, the patient's cognitive performance deteriorated again. With another 1.0 mg of physostygmine it improved once again. The psychiatrist was therefore confident that the OBS was attributable, at least primarily, to anticholinergic toxicity. She also concluded that it would likely improve with further reduction of the amitriptyline and promethazine. She then conferred with the gastroenterologist and rheumatologist, both of whom felt that there was no contraindication to reducing and discontinuing the cimetidine and ibuprofen, at least temporarily. A reduction schedule order for these medications was therefore also written.

Within 48 h the patient's performance on mental status examination revealed no evidence of disturbance in orientation, perception, memory, or thinking, and no disturbed autonomic or psychomotor activity. She was relaxed and optimistic and cooperated fully in her treatment. She continued to have some pain but obtained sufficient relief from acetaminophen. Two days later she was discharged. On subsequent office visits there was no evidence of depression or duodenal ulcer. Her rheumatoid arthritis was managed without nonsteroid anti-inflammatory medications.

Treatment for Specific Causes

Discontinuing medications was sufficient to bring about remission of the OBS in this patient. Had her OBS not been responsive to physostigmine, the psychiatrist, along with her primary physician, would have pursued other less likely causes for the OBS. Many of these, such as endocrine disorders, can be treated effectively and can bring about rapid improvement of OBS. Others, such as cerebral injury or neoplasm, have a less favorable prognosis, but treatment can often be effective in reducing the degree of OBS and patient distress, inability to comply with treatment, and likelihood of accidental injury.

We have outlined a sequence of procedures for recognizing OBS, pursuing possible causes, removing or treating the causes, and treating the symptomatic expressions of OBS pharmacologically and behaviorally. Definitive recognition rests primarily on taking a careful history and conducting a thorough mental status examination. This approach to the patient at risk for OBS can be used readily by all primary physicians. The principles of symptomatic treatment can be understood readily and used effectively by all professional personnel in contact with patients. The use of this approach will increase the likelihood that the significant proportion of physically ill patients with OBS will be diagnosed and treated effectively.

REFERENCES

Bedford, P. D. (1959). General medical aspects of confusional states in elderly people. *British Medical Journal, 2,* 185–188.

Blessed, G., & Wilson, I. D. (1982). The contemporary natural history of mental disorder in old age. *British Journal of Psychiatry, 141,* 59–67.

Butler, R. N. (1978). Overview on aging. In G. Usdin, & C. K. Hofling (Eds.), *Aging: The process and the people.* New York: Brunner/Mazel.

Denny, D., Quass, R. M., & Rich, D. C. (1966). Psychiatric patients on medical wards: Prevalence of illness and recognition of disorders by staff personnel. *Archives of General Psychiatry, 14,* 530–535.

Diagnostic and statistical manual of mental disorders III. (1980). Washington, DC: American Psychiatric Association.

Fishburne, P. M., Abelson, H. I., & Crisin, I. (1980). *National survey on drug abuse: Main findings* (DHHS Publication No. 80–976). Washington, DC: U.S. Government Printing Office.

Guze, S. B., & Cantrell, D. P. (1964). The prognosis in organic brain syndromes. *American Journal of Psychiatry, 120,* 878–881.

Hall, R. C. W., Feinsilver, D. L., & Holt, R. E. (1981). Anticholinergic psychosis: Differential diagnosis and management. *Psychosomatics, 22,* 581–587.

Hendrie, H. C. (1978). Brain disorders: Classification, the "symptomatic" psychoses, misdiagnosis. *The Psychiatric Clinics of North America, 1,* 1–19.

Levin, H. S., & Grossman, R. G. (1978). Behavioral sequelae of closed head injury. *Archives of Neurology, 35,* 720–727.

Lipowski, Z. J. (1980). *Delirium: Acute brain failure in man.* Springfield, IL: Charles C. Thomas.

Lipowski, Z. J. (1983). Transient cognitive disorders (delirium, acute confusional state) in the elderly. *American Journal of Psychiatry, 140,* 1426–1436.

Millar, H. R. (1981). Psychiatric morbidity in elderly surgical patients. *British Journal of Psychiatry, 138,* 17–20.

Penn, J. R., & Mackenzie, T. B. (1983). Organic mental disorder associated with metrizamide. *Psychosomatics, 24,* 849–853.

Preskorn, S. H., & Simpson, S. (1982). Tricyclic antidepressant induced delirium and plasma drug concentration. *American Journal of Psychiatry, 139,* 822–823.

Rabins, P. V., & Folstein, M. F. (1982). Delirium and dementia diagnostic criteria and fatality rates. *British Journal of Psychiatry, 140,* 149–153.

Shevitz, S. A., Silverfarb, P. M., & Lipowski, Z. J. (1976). Psychiatric consultation in a general hospital: A report on 1000 referrals. *Diseases of the Nervous System, 37,* 295–300.

Vestal, R. E. (1978). Drug use in the elderly: A review of problems and special considerations. *Drugs, 16,* 358–382.

Weddington, W. W. (1982). The mortality of delirium: An underappreciated problem? *Psychosomatics, 23,* 1232–1235.

Wells, C. E. (1981). A deluge of dementia. *Psychosomatics, 22,* 837–840.

Chapter 3

THE PSYCHOPHARMACOLOGIC TREATMENT OF PHYSICALLY ILL PATIENTS

C. E. Sermas

Psychotherapeutic interventions alone are often sufficient to aid a patient in emotional distress. However, some patients require more assistance, and psychopharmacologic agents can be of considerable help; in some situations they are the principal therapy. Unfortunately, side effects do exist, some of which can aggravate underlying medical illness; others may create a new disease state such as delirium, interact unfavorably with other medications, harm an unborn child, or intensify the physical frailties of advancing years.

ANTIPSYCHOTICS

Since the recognition of chlorpromazine's efficacy in the treatment of schizophrenic patients, the antipsychotics have become firmly established and widely used agents. Schizophrenia remains the primary indication for the use of antipsychotic drugs, but they are also utilized in treating mania, schizoaffective disorders, psychotic depressions, Tourette's syndrome, dementia-associated psychosis, and delirious states (Hollister, 1978).

Their antipsychotic effects are thought to be related to their ability to block central dopamine receptors, a pharmacologic action that also explains antipsychotic-induced extrapyramidal reactions. These drugs are also alpha-adrenergic blockers and anticholinergics (Van Praag, 1978).

Currently, five classses of antipsychotics are available in the United States: phenothiazine (aliphatic, piperidine, and piperazine), thioxanthene, butyrophenone, hydroxyindolone, and dibenzoxazepine. More practically, if somewhat simply, the antipsychotics can be divided into two groups, the low-potency and high-potency compounds (Zavodnick, 1978). In equivalent antipsychotic doses, the low-potency compounds (chlorpromazine, thioridazine, and chlorprothixene) are more potent anticholinergics, stronger alpha-blockers, more sedating, and generally associated with a wider variety of adverse reactions. The high-potency agents (trifluoperazine, perphenazine, fluphenazine, thiothixene, haloperidol, molindone, and loxapine) are more likely to cause acute extrapyramidal reactions. Mesoridazine can be considered an "intermediate potency" drug (Hollister, 1978; Van Praag, 1978).

Both the low- and high-potency antipsychotics usually are given orally, although members of both groups are available for intramuscular injection. Antipsychotic drugs are thought to be generally well absorbed (Zavodnick, 1978), but intramuscular absorption is more rapid and complete and probably produces plasma concentrations three to four times higher than found with equivalent oral doses. Metabolism is predominantly hepatic, and protein binding is very high (Hollister, 1978).

Generally, the low-potency compounds have been found to have a greater number of active and toxic metabolites than the high-potency agents (Dahl, 1982; Zavodnick, 1978). There is a considerable interindividual variation in plasma concentration. Currently, there is little clinical value in routine plasma-level monitoring, and clinical response is still the best guide to dosage (Van Praag, 1978).

Side Effects

Neurological.   Extrapyramidal syndromes (acute dystonia, akathisia, akinesia, and pseudoparkinsonism) are especially common with the high-potency antipsychotics and quite rare with thioridazine. Treatment with anticholinergics or amantadine is usually effective, and these syndromes tend to disappear with continued antipsychotic therapy. Patients with preexisting Parkinson's disease requiring an antipsychotic might be given thioridazine, but special cautions should be taken to avoid increasing atropinic side effects in those patients already receiving anticholinergic drugs. Because a few cases of drug-induced Parkinson's disease may prove to be quite long-lasting, especially because of the very real risk of tardive dyskinesia, antipsychotic drugs should be used with discretion and even avoided if other psychotropics could be used as effectively (Hollister, 1978).

Antipsychotics also have been associated with hypo- and hyperthermia, reflecting the potential of these drugs to impair centrally mediated mechanisms of thermoregulation. Underlying illness (midbrain disorders, ethanol or barbiturate withdrawal) and extremes of ambient temperature are predisposing factors (Greenblatt, Gross, Harris, Shader, & Circaulo, 1978). Heatstroke, sometimes fatal, has been associated with antipsychotic drugs (Kilbourne, Keewhan, Jones, Thacker, & Field Investigation Team, 1982). The anticholinergic effects of low-potency drugs or coadministration with antiparkinsonism medications would appear to increase the risk. The neuroleptic malignant syndrome (hyperthermia, hypertension, diaphoresis, rigidity, and coma) occurs mainly in young males receiving low-potency agents (Smego & Durack, 1982).

Not surprisingly, sedation and even an atropinic delirium may occur, especially in the brain-compromised or in elderly patients treated with chlorpromazine or thioridazine (Bernstein, 1979). Blurring of vision is a common anticholinergic side effect. Retinitis pigmentosa may occur with high doses of thioridazine (Zavodovnick, 1978). Most cases of glaucoma are of the open-angle type and not aggravated by antipsychotics; in patients with angle-closure glaucoma, drugs with low anticholinergic effects present less risk but should be discontinued if acute eye pain develops (Schwartz, 1978).

The antipsychotics also lower the seizure threshold, as demonstrated in animal studies (Tedeschi, Benigni, Elder, Yeager, & Flanigan, 1958). Information on the effect of antipsychotics on human seizure activity is largely anecdotal, but chlorpromazine appears to be the antipsychotic most commonly associated with epileptiform convulsions. Haloperidol, trifluoperazine, and thioridazine are regarded as the drugs with least effect on the seizure threshold. Although antipsychotic-induced seizures are rare (less than 1 percent of treated patients), a number of factors increase risk: a history of epilepsy, structural brain damage, large or rapidly fluctuating doses, and the prescribing of multiple drugs (Remick & Fine, 1979).

Cardiovascular.   Antipsychotics in therapeutic doses may produce a number of ECG abnormalities, including T-wave changes, ST-segment depression, and widening of the QRS and QT intervals. Thioridazine in particular is associated with a high incidence of such abnormalities. Since a fall in serum potassium tends to bring out these changes, they are more likely to appear after a meal. Fifty-seven percent of these ECG changes reverse after an overnight fast. Those abnormalities that do not normalize generally are associated with low serum potassium and will reverse with administration of potassium or propranolol. Moreover, these ECG abnormalities suggest a quinidine-like effect on myocardial conduction, as is seen with type I antiarrhythmics and tricyclic antidepressants. Baseline and follow-up ECG (during fasting) may help distinguish antipsychotic-induced effects from those reflecting cardiac pathology and those of other medications (Charalampous & Keepers, 1978; Nasrallah, 1978).

Although the ECG changes associated with lower doses of antipsychotics are generally considered benign, at higher and toxic dosages these medications can induce more serious ventricular arrhythmias (ranging from premature ventricular contractions to ventricular tachycardia and fibrillation) through facilitation of reentrant excitation. Varying degrees of heart block also can occur. These adverse reactions are thought to be the cause of sudden death associated with antipsychotics. Although it is difficult to predict which patient will develop such serious complications, the presence of frequent premature ventricular contractions or atrioventricular conduction delays indicates caution (Levenson, Beard, & Murphy, 1980).

Thioridazine is most frequently associated with these problems, followed by chlorpromazine (Charalampous & Keepers, 1978). High-potency agents are less frequently associated with ECG anomalies and sudden death (Zavodnick, 1978).

High-potency antipsychotics also are preferable for patients susceptible to orthostatic hypotension. The relatively high alpha-adrenergic blocking activity of chlorpromazine and thioridazine presents a particular risk to patients with coronary artery of cerebrovascular disease, especially if they are receiving vasodilators (Bernstein, 1979).

Animal studies suggest that high doses of thioridazine depress myocardial contractility, heart rate, cardiac output, and coronary blood flow. Thus, some care should be taken in giving antipsychotic medications to patients with myocardial compromise and those patients who will be engaged in vigorous physical exercise (Nasrallah, 1978).

Respiratory.   Generally, toxic amounts of antipsychotic drugs are required to suppress respiratory effort severely. If muscular spasms caused by antipsychotic overdose are mistaken for seizure activity, the administration of anticonvulsants can potentiate respiratory depression (Hollister, 1978). When treating patients with diminished respiratory capacity, thioridazine and chlorpromazine should be used carefully or even avoided because of their sedative effects. Acute laryngeal spasm, which responds to anticholinergic medication, has been associated with haloperidol (Flaherty & Lahmeyer, 1978). A respiratory dyskinesia manifested by shortness of breath, irregular breathing, respiratory alkalosis, diminished arterial oxygen tension, and classical signs of tardive dyskinesia also has been described (Jamm & Bitar, 1982).

Gastrointestinal.   Antipsychotics frequently have been used to control nausea and vomiting. Generally, the piperazines have the greatest antiemetic effect, whereas thioridazine does not demonstrate this property. Chlorpromazine is employed in the treatment of hiccups. Their effects are beneficial, but there is a risk that antipsychotics can mask the development of serious gastrointestinal symptoms (Van Praag, 1978).

Because of their anticholinergic effects, antipsychotic medications can cause delayed gastric emptying, constipation, fecal impaction, and even paralytic ileus (Hollister, 1978). The higher-potency agents are less likely to decrease bowel motility.

Hepatic.   Although antipsychotics are not contraindicated in patients with liver disease, they are predominantly metabolized hepatically. Lower and less frequent doses can help reduce the danger of overdose (Strain, 1975).

Occasionally, the antipsychotics have been associated with cholestatic jaundice, manifested by fever, hepatic tenderness, and anorexia. Serum bilirubin and alkaline phosphatase are elevated, and biopsy reveals little parenchymal damage. Chlorpromazine is most commonly implicated, whereas thioridazine and trifluoperazine are thought to carry the least risk. Since this reaction occurs early in treatment and is accompanied by eosinophilia, it is thought to be an allergic response. Discontinuation of the offending agent reverses the problem, and another neuroleptic can usually be given without difficulty (Charalampous & Keepers, 1978; Strain, 1975). Very rarely, a xanthomatous biliary cirrhosis may ensue (Devaris & Mehlman, 1979).

Renal.   Generally, the high-potency antipsychotics are preferable to the low-potency agents in the treatment of patients with renal failure. Chlorpromazine and thioridazine are more likely to aggravate the blood pressure fluctuations that patients with renal compromise are especially prone to experience. Also, accumulation of toxic metabolites is more likely with the low-potency antipsychotics. Strain (1975) has recommended trifluoperazine for patients with renal failure, cautioning that the dosage should be reduced by half in moderate failure and by two-thirds in the face of severe renal failure.

Metabolic/Endocrine.   Increased appetite with secondary weight gain is commonly seen with antipsychotic medications. Impaired glucose tolerance also has been reported. This problem may represent reduced effective insulin available secondary to phenothiazine-induced obesity or possibly a direct inhibition of insulin release in prediabetics. Antipsychotics also inhibit the dopamine-mediated inhibition of prolactin release and can cause galactorrhea in female patients. Women treated with antipsychotics also may experience amenorrhea; some male patients develop gynecomastia (Charalampous & Keepers, 1978; Van Praag, 1978).

As the antipsychotics are strongly protein-bound (Hollister, 1978), dosages given debilitated, hypoproteinemic patients should be small, since the unbound "active" medication fraction may be relatively increased. Conservative dosages also are indicated for hypothyroid patients, since their ability to metabolize these very potent medications may be severely attenuated; phenothiazine-induced hypothermic coma has been reported in such cases (Devaris & Mehlman, 1979).

Hematologic.   Although quite unusual, thrombopenia and thrombopenic purpura, hemolytic anemias, and pancytopenia have been associated with antipsychotic medications. These conditions generally reverse with elimination of the offensive agent, and another antipsychotic usually can be substituted (Hollister, 1964).

Angranulocytosis occurs in less than 1 percent of patients receiving antipsychotics, usually during the first few weeks of therapy, and can prove fatal. Most cases involve older white women, often obese and in poor health, exposed to low-potency agents, particularly chlorpromazine (Charalampous & Keepers, 1978), and the declining incidence of this serious side effect in recent years may reflect increasing usage of higher-potency agents (Ducomb & Baldessarini, 1977). The onset of fever, sore throat, and adenopathy during the first 12 weeks of therapy with any antipsychotic should be considered a possible indicator of agranulocytosis.

Geriatric.   Older patients are generally more sensitive to a number of antipsychotic medication side effects, including orthostatic hypotension, sedation, anticholinergic reactions, and cardiotoxicity. Attenuated metabolism and excretion of most psychotropic drugs, together with a higher prevalence of hypertension, arteriosclerotic cerebrovascular and coronary artery disease, and organic brain disease in the geriatric population, dictates cautious administration of medications as potent as the antipsychotic drugs. The low-potency antipsychotics (chlorpromazine and thioridazine) are considerably more sedating, more frequently associated with serious cardiotoxicity, higher in anticholinergic activity, and more prone to cause orthostatic hypotension than the high-potency agents. Increased pulse rate can lower ventricular filling time and thus decrease cardiac output, risking the onset or worsening of congestive heart failure. Hypotension in the face of arteriosclerotic cerebrovascular disease carries an increased risk of stroke or transient ischemic attack. Anticholinergic effects in patients with prostatic enlargement could lead to urinary retention. Therefore, when antipsychotic therapy is indicated for an older patient, the high-potency drugs generally present less risk of serious side effects (Bernstein, 1979; Neshkes & Jarvik, 1982; Salzman, 1982; Zavodnick, 1978).

Pregnancy and Breast Feeding.   As with other psychotropic drugs, antipsychotics enter the fetal circulation and should not be administered to pregnant women for trivial reasons, especially during the first trimester. The drugs can be useful for treatment of hyperemesis gravidarum and severe psychiatric disturbances arising during pregnancy. Case reports have associated antipsychotics with spontaneous abortion, stillbirths, and a variety of congenital malformations. However, controlled studies have not supported these concerns. Infants born to mothers given fairly large doses of antipsychotics late in pregnancy have shown a variety of generally reversible neonatal problems, including jaundice, extrapyramidal reaction (sometimes prolonged), apathy, hypotonia, and respiratory distress (Goldberg & DiMascio, 1978).

Fortunately, when an expectant mother's emotional status dictates that the fetus also be exposed to antipsychotic drugs, the risks to fetus and newborn seem to be relatively low. Currently, the clinical question of whether mothers treated with antipsychotics should avoid breast feeding their newborn is rather cloudy. All antipsychotics probably appear in human breast milk, apparently at low concentrations. Observations of the human situation has revealed no overt developmental problems in newborns receiving antipsychotics through breast feeding (Ananth, 1978). Conversely, elegant animal data suggest that dopaminergic neurons undergo important development in the first few weeks postpartum and that antipsychotics given to nursing mothers in low doses hinders the development of these dopamine-dependent pathways, leading to significant compromise in accomplishing new learning tasks (Lundborg & Engel, 1978). However, the clinical pertinence of "behavioral teratogenicity" remains unclear.

Drug-Drug Interactions.   All antipsychotic drugs are anticholinergic to some degree, particularly chlorpromazine and thioridazine. Concurrent administration of other anticholinergics (antiparkinsonism drugs, antihistamines, tricyclic antidepressants, and so forth) increase the probability that patients will develop dry mouth, blurring of vision, constipation, fecal impaction, and excessive sedation, or more serious anticholinergic complications, such as dental caries, exacerbation of angle-closure glaucoma, ileus, toxic delirium, or urinary retention. The low-potency drugs are also more potent alpha-adrenergic blockers than are the high-potency antipsychotics and are therefore more likely to cause orthostatic hypotension (Zavodnick, 1978). The risk of significant hypotension increases with the addition of beta-blockers, which can hinder compensatory tachycardia. Not surprisingly, vasodilators also can enhance the hypotensive effects of antipsychotic drugs (Dahl, 1982; Hollister, 1978; Van Praag, 1978).

Similar to tricyclic antidepressants, chlorpromazine (and perhaps thiothixine and haloperidol) may antagonize the hypotensive effects of guanethidine by blocking its neuronal uptake. Thus, a severe hypotension could ensue if guanethidine dosage is increased and the antipsychotic is suddenly withdrawn (Sandifer, 1978).

When antipsychotics and tricyclic antidepressants are used together, each drug appears to inhibit the metabolism and increase serum concentrations of the other. Chlorpromazine (and perhaps other antipsychotics) can enhance lithium elimination. Moreover, haloperidol in combination with lithium has been associated with severe extrapyramidal reactions and irreversible encephalopathy. Monoamine oxidase (MAO) inhibitors have been reported to inhibit metabolism of antipsychotic drugs, and the combination also may increase the probability of a hypotensive episode (Gualtieri & Powell, 1978).

Antipsychotic medications also have a type I antiarrhythmic effect. Combination with quinidine, procainamide, and disopyramide can lead to signs of quinidine toxicity (Levenson et al., 1980).

Phenytoin metabolism may be reduced by antipsychotics, especially chlorpromazine; therefore, phenytoin toxicity can be enhanced. Prolonged administration of another anticonvulsant, phenobarbital, may increase chlorpromazine metabolism (Gualtieri & Powell, 1978).

ANTIDEPRESSANTS

Antidepressant drugs are divided into two chemical groups: the tricyclic antidepressants (TCA) and monoamine oxidase inhibitors (MAOI). Recently, "second generation" antidepressants have been introduced into clinical use.

The TCA group can be divided into the tertiary amines (imipramine, amitriptyline, doxepin) and the secondary amines (desipramine, nortriptyline, protriptyline). Congruent with the amine hypothesis of depression, all block central presynaptic reuptake of norepinephrine and/or serotonin (Hollister, 1978; Van Praag, 1978), although their overall efficacy in ameliorating symptoms of major depressive disorders also may depend on modulation of the sensitivity of alpha- and beta-adrenergic receptors (Bernstein, 1978).

The tertiary amines have more sedative and anticholinergic properties and more influence on serotonin reuptake than do the secondary amines, which tend to block norepinephrine reuptake (Hollister, 1978). TCA are more effective in major depressive disorders than in neurotic depressions (Van Praag, 1978). They also have been used in the treatment of panic states and phobic anxiety (Klein, Zitrin, & Woerner, 1978), narcolepsy (Regenstein, Reich, & Mufson, 1983), sleep apnea (Clark, Schmidt, Schaal, Boudoulas, & Schuller, 1979) and migraine headaches and other painful conditions (Hollister, 1978).

Amitriptyline and imipramine are available in injectable form for intramuscular use, but TCA are generally given orally. Gastrointestinal absorption is complete, metabolism is hepatic, and protein-binding is quite high (Hollister, 1978.) Actual plasma concentrations vary greatly between individuals and show some correlation with therapeutic effect, especially for imipramine and nortriptyline, and to some degree for amitriptyline. TCA plasma levels generally are not recommended for routine clinical use but are of great potential benefit for patients who do not respond to seemingly adequate doses, patients who may be vulnerable to severe adverse reactions to TCA, and patients whose metabolism of TCA may be affected by illness and/or other medications (Gramm, Pederson, Kristensen, & Kraugh-Sorensen, 1982).

The MAOI also can be divided into two groups, the hydrazide (phenelzine) and nonhydrazide (tranylcypromine, isocarboxazide, pargyline). Pargyline is used as an antihypertensive, whereas the remaining compounds usually are reserved for major depressive disorders refractory to TCA therapy. Some literature indicates that MAOI may be very effective in treatment of neurotic or "atypical" depressive disorders (Liebowitz et al., 1981) and possibly panic states and phobias (Klein et al., 1978).

Currently available MAOI inhibit both MAO type A and MAO type B. MAO type A utilizes norepinephrine, dopamine, and serotonin as substrates, and MAOI increase concentrations of these amines in the brain (Hollister, 1978). Like TCA, MAOI are administered orally and metabolized by the liver. Plasma levels probably are not useful, but therapeutic effect does appear to correlate with 80 percent or greater suppression of platelet MAO activity (Van Praag, 1978).

Among the newer antidepressants, trimipramine is a true TCA with efficacy and adverse reactions similar to the more established agents (Rifkin, Saraf, Kane, Ross, & Klein, 1980). Amoxapine is chemically related to the antipsychotic loxapine and blocks postsynaptic dopamine receptors; fewer side effects than with amitriptyline have been claimed. Maprotiline is a tetracyclic compound with a secondary amine side chain and therapeutic action (inhibition of norepinephrine reuptake) and side effects similar to desipramine. Trazodone is a triazolopyridine that blocks serotonin reuptake, much like amitriptyline. It seems to possess few, if any, anticholinergic side effects and is reportedly less cardiotoxic than TCA. Alprazolam, a benzodiazepine with a triazolo ring in its structure, shows some promise in the treatment of depressive states. The full benefits and risks associated with these newer agents are, as of now, undetermined (Hollister, 1981b).

Side Effects

Neurological. Oversedation and frank confusional states can be caused by TCA, especially in older patients. The risk increases when other sedating medications, particularly anticholinergics, are coadministered. TCA also can aggravate essential tremor or cause a similar tremor as a side effect; in either case propranolol can be helpful. TCA can diminish parkinsonian tremor, but other anticholinergics should be reduced or discontinued when TCA are given. Blurring of vision is a common anticholinergic side effect. TCA do lower the seizure threshold but are not contraindicated in well-controlled epilepsy. Patients with underlying brain damage are probably most vulnerable to TCA-induced seizures (Bernstein, 1979; Hollister, 1978; Van Praag, 1978).

Because they are anticholinergic, TCA may aggravate narrow-angle glaucoma. Such reactions are infrequent when the glaucoma is well controlled. Open-angle glaucoma presents no problem (Schwartz, 1978). MAOI are not particularly anticholinergic and appear to have little effect on the seizure threshold (Bernstein, 1978).

Cardiovascular. Both TCA and MAOI can produce significant cardiovascular effects, especially in patients with preexisting cardiovascular disease (Robinson & Barker, 1976). Although antidepressant pharmacotherapy is not necessarily contraindicated in such individuals, the use of MAOI and TCA or related drugs requires respectful caution.

Orthostatic hypotension is the most common serious side effect of antidepressant treatment and has been associated with virtually all available agents. This problem has been most widely studied among the TCA, which probably cause this problem by centrally inhibiting vasomotor tone (Hayes, Born, & Rosenbaum, 1977). Orthostatic hypotension tends to appear early in TCA treatment at subtherapeutic blood levels, does not worsen with therapeutic dosage increments, and does not improve with reduction of TCA dose.

Nortriptyline seems to have less of an adverse action on postural blood pressure than other TCA. Whereas any patient with significant debilitation receiving TCA or MAOI should have regular supine and standing determinations of blood pressure, patients with arteriosclerotic coronary artery or cerebrovascular disease may be at special risk, since hypotension and resultant fall in perfusion could lead to myocardial infarction, ischemia-induced arrhythmia, transient ischemic attack, or stroke (Davidson & Wenger, 1982).

TCA tend to increase pulse rate in most individuals. Amitriptyline may cause as much as 20 percent rise in heart rate; less anticholinergic drugs (desipramine, nortriptyline) have less effect on pulse (Davidson & Wenger, 1982). Trazodone, claimed to have no anticholinergic properties, has not been associated with increased heart rate but does cause hypotension (Risch & Janowsky, 1981). MAOI actually may cause a decrease in pulse rate (Davidson & Wenger, 1982).

TCA may have more affinity for cardiac than skeletal muscle, and effects on cardiac conduction and myocardial contractility are of concern. Probably the most common ECG abnormality associated with therapeutic doses of TCA is nonspecific T-wave changes; prolongation of the PR and QRS intervals also have been noted (Bigger, Kantor, Glassman, & Perel, 1978). In toxic doses TCA have been associated with a number of serious arrhythmias, most commonly conduction defects (atrioventricular, bundle branch, and intraventricular blocks) (Hollister, 1981b).

Normally, the sinoatrial node generates an electrical impulse that is rapidly transmitted via three atrial tracts to the atrioventricular node (AVN), where conduction slows and is vulnerable to block. From the AVN the impulse is carried to the ventricles through the ventricular specialized conduction system (VSCS) composed of the bundle of His and its two branches, the right and left bundles, and finally, the distal Purkinje fibers. The TCA-associated prolongation of PR and QRS intervals appears to represent depression of VSCS activity, similar to the effects of type I antiarrhythmics (quinidine, procainamide, and disopyramide) (Bigger et al., 1978). Clinically, these findings seem to correlate with the observation that TCA, like quinidine, tend to decrease the frequency of premature ventricular and atrial contractions. Although these quinidine-like effects are therapeutic in cases of cardiac irritability, patients with bundle branch block or some other form of conduction delay are at risk of worsening during TCA therapy. Amitriptyline and imipramine are probably most likely to depress VSCS function (Davidson & Wenger, 1982). Nortriptyline at therapeutic plasma levels appears less likely to cause these difficulties (Bigger et al., 1978). Doxepin also has been recommended, but its effects on cardiac conduction at therapeutic levels is less established. MAOI actually may shorten PR and QT intervals and probably can be used safely in patients with known conduction impairment (Davidson & Wenger, 1982).

The effects of TCA on myocardial contractility are less known than their effect on cardiac conduction. Animal studies indicate that low doses of imipramine have a positive ionotropic effect, whereas higher doses result in reduced myocardial performance (Muller, Goodman, & Bellet, 1961). Congestive failure has been reported as a complication of TCA therapy and overdose, and patients with preexisting cardiovascular disease generally are considered to be at greater risk (Jefferson, 1975). However, in one study imipramine was used successfully in patients with healed myocardial infarcts (Raskind, Vieth, Barnes, & Gumbrecht, 1982), and in another imipramine and doxepin were used effectively in depressed patients with known cardiovascular disease without effect on left ventricular ejection fraction at rest or during maximal exercise as measured by radionucleotide ventriculograms (Vieth et al., 1982). Noninvasive measures of ventricular function, such as radionucleotide ventriculography or M-mode echocardiography, together with ECG and TCA plasma-level determinations, may reduce the risk of myocardial decompensation in vulnerable patients (Murburg, Anton, Nelson, & Atlow, 1982). Although interagent dif ferences have not been established for TCA, agents with low anticholinergic activity (desipramine, nortriptyline) have been recommended for depressed patients prone to congestive heart failure.

As alternative agents MAOI appear to increase myocardial contractility and coronary blood flow (Davidson & Wenger, 1982). Newer tricyclic, tetracyclic, and novel medication may have fewer cardiotoxic effects, but further clinical evaluation is necessary (Hollister, 1981b). Antidepressant drug therapy should be avoided in overt congestive heart failure and during the first 3 months following myocardial infarction.

Respiratory.   Because TCA are sedating, they can reduce respiratory drive. However, substantial overdose is required to produce any significant clinical effect, and sudden apnea is a reported complication of TCA overdosage (Hollister, 1978). The more sedating TCA should be used cautiously in patients with compromised respiratory function. When physostigmine, a drug with cholinergic effects, is used in the management of TCA overdose, underlying reactive airway disease can be aggravated (Granacher & Baldessarini, 1975).

Gastrointestinal.   The gastrointestinal effects of TCA are mainly anticholinergic. Constipation and fecal impaction can occur; adynamic ileus is also possible and potentially fatal. Relaxation of the esophageal sphincter can symptomatically aggravate hiatus hernia (Hollister, 1978; Van Praag, 1978). TCA, particularly amitriptyline, doxepin, and trimipramine block histaminic-2 receptors that stimulate parietal cell production of gastric acid. TCA may prove to be as potent as cimetidine in reducing gastric acidity (Jagdish & Pereira, 1982).

Hepatic.   Both TCA and MAOI have been associated with cholestatic jaundice; this is probably an allergic reaction similar to that with antipsychotic drugs. Discontinuation of the offending drug usually will reverse the problem. Moderate rises of hepatic enzymes, particularly alkaline phosphatase and the transaminases, are common during TCA therapy. A few cases of fatal hepatic necrosis have been associated with various TCA (Blackwell, 1981).

The presence of hepatic dysfunction does not necessarily contraindicate the use of antidepressants. However, both TCA and MAOI are hepatically metabolized, so that lower than usual dosage may prove therapeutic and help avoid toxicity. In such situations monitoring of TCA plasma levels may be of particular utility.

Renal. Imipramine and amitriptyline, the prototypical TCA, are completely metabolized by hepatic mechanisms, and generally neither drug requires dosage reduction in the presence of renal failure (Bennett, Singer & Coggins, 1970). Desipramine and nortriptyline offer the same metabolic advantage and would seem less likely to induce hypotension, sedation, cardiac disturbances, and other side effects that patients with renal dysfunction may be particularly prone to develop.

Metabolic/Endocrine. Weight gain is well associated with antidepressant medication therapy with both TCA and MAOI. A subjective craving for sweets has been noted in patients treated with amitriptyline (Bennet, Singer & Coggins, 1970; Hollister, 1978). Some authors caution that TCA have a slight antidiabetic effect that could necessitate adjustments in dosage of medications given to control diabetes (Van Praag, 1978). Others cite studies indicating that TCA have no effect on glucose tolerance or insulin levels (Hollister, 1978; Bennett, Singer & Coggins, 1970). MAOI occasionally have been associated with hypoglycemia and peripheral edema (Bennett, Singer, & Coggins, 1970). Galactorrhea also has been cited as an adverse effect of TCA therapy. However, only amoxapine, an antidepressant agent structurally related to the antipsychotic loxapine, has been clearly associated with elevated prolactin levels and galactorrhea; not surprisingly, amoxapine also causes menstrual irregularities similar to those seen with antipsychotic drugs (Cooper, D.S. et al., 1981).

Hematologic. Rare case reports have associated TCA

treatment with nonthrombocytopenic purpura. TCA also have been implicated as a possible cause of agranulocytosis (Blackwell, 1981). Fortunately, this reaction seems even less frequent with the TCA than with the antipsychotic drugs. As with the antipsychotics, older females appear to be more vulnerable. However, the latency period (initiation of drug to onset of symptoms) is longer and recovery more rapid in cases of TCA-associated agranulocytosis (Albertini & Penders, 1978).

Geriatric. As with the antipsychotic drugs, older patients are more sensitive to a variety of TCA side effects, especially sedation, anticholinergic effects (including delirium and urinary retention), orthostatic hypotension, and cardiotoxicity. Age is correlated with increased TCA plasma half-life, and severe toxicity can occur at seemingly low dosages. The hypotensive effects of both TCA and MAOI are of particular concern in the face of increased incidence of arteriosclerotic cerebrovascular and coronary artery disease in the geriatric population. Hypoperfusion of the cerebral vasculature can lead to transient ischemic attacks and stroke. Hypotension also can reduce coronary artery blood flow, risking ischemia-induced arrythmias or myocardial infarct (Salzman, 1982; Strain, 1975).

Pregnancy and Breast Feeding. Isolated case reports have associated both imipramine and amitriptyline, used during pregnancy, with congenital malformations. Larger series of patients and controlled studies have failed to demonstrate any significant association between TCA and birth defects. Although reassuring, such results do not condone the cavalier use of these powerful agents during early pregnancy. Similarly, ingestion of TCA during the third trimester has been associated occasionally with neonatal hypotonia, respiratory distress, muscular spasms, and urinary retention, apparently without long-term sequelae (Goldberg & DiMascio, 1978).

Imipramine, desipramine, amitriptyline, and the MAOI tranylcypromine have been detected in human breast milk but in such exceedingly small amounts that both TCA and MAOI generally have been regarded as safe drugs for nursing mothers (Ananth, 1978). Generally, little is known about the effects of second-generation antidepressants on pregnancy, fetal development, and breast feeding.

Drug-Drug Interactions.   TCA, particularly the tertiary amines, have a sedative effect. Therefore, combination with other central nervous system depressants (hypnotics, low-potency antipsychotics, opiates, benzodiazepines, general anesthesia, and so forth) can produce additive sedative effects. Since TCA are also anticholinergic, their concurrent administration with other anticholinergics increases the chance of troublesome anticholinergic reactions (Gualtieri & Powell, 1978; Hollister, 1978).

TCA can inhibit the metabolism of stimulants (amphetamine, methylphenidate); the metabolism of TCA may be diminished by methylphenidate-induced inhibition of hydroxylating enzymes, leading to increased TCA serum concentration. Concurrent use of an antipsychotic and TCA tends to increase serum concentrations of both compounds, perhaps because both drugs are metabolized through the cytochrome P450 system (Annitto, Prien, & Gershon, 1980). Conversely, barbiturates, meprobamate, alcohol, and nicotine may induce hepatic enzymes that metabolize TCA, causing decreased TCA serum levels and perhaps loss of therapeutic effect. Similarly, methaqualone, glutethimide, chloral hydrate, and diphenhydramine are thought to lower TCA plasma concentration (Gualtieri & Powell, 1978; Siris & Rifkin, 1981).

Antihypertensive medications, principally reserpine and to a lesser extent methyldopa and propranolol, have been associated with depressive symptoms. Assuming that antihypertensive therapy alone is not the cause of a patient's depression, some possible drug interactions are important to consider. TCA block the antihypertensive effects of guanethidine. In addition, abrupt discontinuation of TCA can lead to sudden and excessive guanethidine-induced hypotension. TCA also inhibit the antihypertensive effect of clonidine. Although TCA have been postulated to interfere with the antihypertensive action of methyldopa, the combination of the two drugs is generally compatible. TCA do not significantly alter the antihypertensive effects of diuretics, propranolol, or hydralazine (Sandifer, 1978), but the risk of orthostatic hypotension is increased.

The pressor effects of epinephrine, norepinephrine, and phenylephrine are considerably potentiated by TCA (Sandifer, 1978; Van Praag, 1978). Because TCA have a type I antiarrhythmic effect, they can potentiate the actions of quinidine, procainamide, and disopyramide (Blackwell, 1981). TCA also have been cited as possible inhibitors of dicoumarol metabolism but probably do not appreciably affect the metabolism of warfarin (Gualtieri & Powell, 1978; Strain, 1975).

As with antipsychotic drugs, the MAOI cause orthostatic hypotension that may be aggravated by vasodilators and beta-blockers. The risk of hypertensive crisis from the combination of MAOI with sympathomimetic compounds is well known. Usually these pressor responses are mild but can be very serious. In combination with MAOI, large amounts of caffeine or chocolate, tyramine-rich foods and beverages (aged cheese, pickled herring, chicken livers, red wine, and sherry), amphetamines, methylphenidate, and phenylephrine may significantly increase blood pressure. The pressor effects of isoproterenol, epinephrine, and norepinephrine may not be potentiated by MAOI, but caution is advisable. Although TCA and MAOI have been used together in the treatment of refractory depressions, the combination does carry the risk of hypertension (Blackwell, 1981; Hollister, 1978; Van Praag, 1978). The anticonvulsant carbamazepine is structurally related to the TCA, and combination with MAOI may present similar risk.

Perhaps through the inhibition of hepatic enzymes, MAOI may potentiate the central nervous system depressant effects of alcohol, barbiturates, benzodiazepines, opiates (especially meperidine), and general anesthetics. MAOI also may enhance the hypotensive effects of spinal anesthetics and prolong the muscle relaxant effects of succinylcholine (Gualtieri & Powell, 1978). When possible, it would seem prudent to discontinue MAOI therapy at least a week before surgery.

Currently, little is known about interactions between second-generation antidepressants and other medications. Since these newer compounds are generally similar to the tricyclics, similar drug interactions might be anticipated.

LITHIUM

Structurally, the lithium ion is the simplest of psychotropic agents, yet lithium has been therapeutically utilized in a variety of disorders. Lithium is the drug of choice in the treatment of acute mania and hypomania and also provides prophylaxis against recurrence of these affective states. The exact mechanism of action remains unknown; but consistent with the amine hypothesis of affective disorders, lithium appears to reduce the amount of norepinephrine and serotonin at central postsynaptic receptors, probably through an inhibition of release and enhancement of reuptake. Together with these antimanic effects, it seems clear that lithium also is effective in the treatment and prophylaxis of bipolar depressive episodes. Additionally, there is evidence that lithium is effective as an antidepressant and as prophylactic medication for recurrent unipolar depressive disorders (Hollister, 1978; Van Praag, 1978). Lithium also may have therapeutic effects in schizophrenia, schizoaffective disorders, emotionally unstable character disorder, recurring inappropriate aggression, alcoholism with evidence of depression, organic brain syndromes with unstable mood, and cluster headaches (Annitto et al., 1980).

Lithium is available only for oral administration in tablet, capsule, and liquid form. Absorption is complete within 6–8 h, with peak plasma levels occurring within 30 min to 2 h after ingestion. There is no protein binding or hepatic metabolism. CSF levels peak 24 h after plasma levels, and the shift into brain tissue is relatively slow. Plasma half-life is about 20 h; lithium is eliminated through the kidney at a rate of about 20 percent of the creatinine clearance, although there can be considerable interindividual variation.

Steady-state plasma concentrations generally occur at about 5 days. In the acute treatment situation, plasma concentration of 0.9 to 1.4 mEq/L are generally required. Maintenance levels of 0.6 to 1.0 mEq/L are usually sufficient for prophylaxis in affective disorders. Because dosage requirements vary and because lithium toxicity is almost always apparent at plasma concentrations of 2.0 mEq/L, monitoring of plasma levels is important until a steady state is reached and during maintenance therapy (Hollister, 1978).

Recently, long-acting lithium preparations have been introduced. Steady-state levels are not appreciably different from traditional forms of lithium, with the added advantage of greater convenience to the patient and possible reduction of peak-related side effects (Cooper, T. B., Simpson, Lee, & Bergner, 1978).

Side Effects

Neurological.   A variety of neurological effects has been associated with lithium therapy. Organic mental disorders are not surprising at toxic levels, but confusional states (often with lethargy, ataxia, and dysarthria) have been reported at modest to low lithium levels. The EEG is usually abnormal, and there is often evidence of some degree of preexisting cerebral dysfunction (Ghadirian & Lehmann, 1980). Although lithium has been used successfully in cerebrally compromised individuals, baseline EEG, minimum therapeutic levels, and periodic reassessment of cognition would seem prudent.

Relatively well controlled epilepsy is not a contraindication to lithium therapy, and some reports indicate that lithium may suppress epileptic seizures and improve interictal behavior (Gershon & Yuwiler, 1960). Yet focal and generalized seizures do occur with severe lithium toxicity and seizures (grand mal and psychomotor) have been associated with therapeutic levels of lithium. Seizure-prone individuals, including those with a history of childhood febrile convulsions or Guillain-Barré syndrome, are probably at greater risk for seizures provoked by therapeutic levels of lithium (Demers, Lukesh, & Prichard, 1970).

Lithium has some neuromuscular effects. A small percentage of treated patients may evidence cogwheeling rigidity that seems generally unresponsive to benztropine mesylate. Lithium is not contraindicated in parkinsonism, but this effect should be kept in mind. More frequently, lithium causes a mild to moderate fine tremor, which may respond to propranolol therapy

(Kane, Rifkin, Quitkin, & Klein, 1978). Transient muscle weakness is common in early stages of lithium therapy. More seriously, lithium may aggravate myasthenia gravis. Since lithium may decrease the presynaptic synthesis and release of acetylcholine, extreme caution should be exercised in giving lithium to patients with neuromuscular disorders or those who receive neuromuscular blocking agents during surgery or electroconvulsive therapy (ECT) (Neil, Himmelhoch, & Licata, 1976).

Cardiovascular. That patients receiving therapeutic dosages of lithium can manifest ECG changes, generally T-wave flattening or inversion, is well established. This finding was once thought to be relatively infrequent. More sophisticated monitoring has demonstrated that perhaps all lithium-treated patients can be expected to show T-wave changes (Demers & Henniger, 1971). These T-wave abnormalities generally appear during the first few weeks of therapy and persist with continued treatment. The T-wave abnormalities disappear after lithium is eliminated from the body. These benign changes are thought to result from a partial displacement of potassium from the myocardium caused by lithium, even if plasma potassium levels are normal (Singer & Rotenberg, 1973).

Tilkian, Schroeder, Kao, and Hultgren (1976) studied cardiovascular performance in 12 patients before and after lithium treatment. Eight patients were known to have some form of cardiovascular abnormality. Lithium had no effect on exercise tolerance and tended to decrease premature atrial contractions. Three patients did have premature ventricular contractions (one case with couplets), leading to a conclusion that lithium may aggravate ventricular arrhythmias.

Isolated cases of arrhythmias have been associated with therapeutic lithium levels, often in patients with preexisting cardiac problems or those taking other, possibly cardiotoxic drugs. Reports have included ventricular tachycardia and fibrillation, multiple premature ventricular contractions, sinus node dysfunction, sinoatrial block, and atrioventricular irritability. Lithium also may dampen atrial impulse generation and transmission and impede atrioventricular conduction. Lithium also has been associated with two cases of myocarditis. There has been little association with myocardial infarction, and lithium has even been used successfully on an emergency basis during post-infarct recovery (Mitchell & Mackenzie, 1982).

In congestive heart failure, diminished renal perfusion decreases lithium clearance, resulting in possible toxicity. Similarly, salt restriction causes increased lithium retention. Factors interfering with lithium excretion should be identified and lithium dosage adjusted accordingly.

Respiratory.   In therapeutic doses lithium is not particularly sedating. However, patients with severe lithium toxicity may require respiratory assistance.

Gastrointestinal.   A variety of gastrointestinal disturbances, including pain, nausea, vomiting, bloating, gastric irritation, anorexia, and diarrhea, often accompany the initiation of lithium therapy. These symptoms generally reflect rapidly rising serum lithium levels and usually can be attenuated by more gradual dosage increases (Reisberg & Gershon, 1979). The presence of severe gastrointestinal symptoms in a patient previously stabilized on therapeutic doses of lithium should alert the clinician to possible lithium toxicity, secondary to dehydration, sodium loss, or some other mechanism.

Hepatic.   The liver plays no significant role in lithium metabolism. Lithium does not appear to be associated with any particular hepatic side effects.

Renal.   About one-half of patients initiating lithium treatment develop a vasopressin-resistant diabetes-insipidus-like syndrome, manifested as polyuria, polydipsia, low urinary specific gravity, and an inability to concentrate urine. This effect may persist in about one-quarter of patients and is generally benign. Thiazide diuretics may help alleviate these symptoms but should be used with caution (Reisberg & Gershon, 1979).

Renal compromise is not an absolute contraindication to lithium therapy. Since lithium is cleared almost entirely by the kidney, dosage increments should be very deliberate, and close monitoring is of extreme importance. Certain diuretics and sodium restriction increase the risk of toxicity; therefore the diuretic regimen should be stabilized before lithium treatment begins.

Zetin, Plon, Nosratola, Cramer, and Greco (1981) reported the successful administration of lithium carbonate to three chronic hemodialysis patients. The patients received a single dose of lithium after each dialysis treatment, and levels were monitored weekly prior to a dialysis treatment. Initial doses were small (300 mg), and a dose of 600 mg achieved therapeutic blood levels.

In recent years some reports have associated chronic lithium therapy with the onset of renal insufficiency accompanied by interstitial nephritis. Although most of these studies can be cited for a variety of inherent shortcomings, the possibility of irreversible lithium-induced renal damage is cause for concern. Careful evaluation of renal functioning prior to lithium therapy, plus periodic reassessment, has been prudently suggested (Ramsey & Cox, 1982).

Metabolic/Endocrine.   A number of reports have asserted that lithium may have an insulin-like effect, possibly by blocking cyclic adenosine monophosphate (AMP)–mediated gluconeogenesis and glucose release from the liver. This may explain the weight gain observed in about one-third of patients on long-term lithium therapy. Caloric restriction, without unnecessary sodium or fluid restriction, will generally control the problem (Reisberg & Gershon, 1979). Lithium is not contraindicated in stable diabetes mellitus.

Lithium does have an antithyroid effect. An enhanced thyroid-stimulating hormone (TSH) response to thyrotropin-releasing hormone may be the only detectable abnormality. Few patients develop goiter or symptomatic hypothyroidism. If these problems develop, thyroid supplement is usually sufficient; if not, lithium discontinuation reverses the abnormalities. Pretreatment TSH, T4, and T3 levels are recommended, with periodic thyroid palpation and monitoring of TSH levels (Hollister, 1978; Van Praag, 1978). Thyroid disturbance is not a contraindication to lithium therapy, but patients with preexisting thyroiditis may be especially vulnerable to the rapid onset of lithium-provoked hypothyroidism.

In a controlled study, Franks et al. (1982) demonstrated elevated levels of total calcium, ionized calcium, and parathyroid hormone in patients undergoing chronic lithium therapy. Although the elevations were modest, the author suggested total calcium, ionized calcium, albumin, and possibly parathyroid determinations for lithium-treated patients who develop disturbances (affective symptoms, hypertension, kidney stones, or renal disease) that could be caused by hypercalcemia.

Hematologic. Most patients receiving lithium treatment evidence a relative leukocytosis, principally a neutrophilia. White blood cell counts rise on average into the 14,000-to-15,000/mm³ range and return to pretreatment levels after lithium discontinuation. The leukocytosis may persist or occur episodically during treatment (Reisberg & Gershon, 1979). Although those changes appear benign, caution should be taken in interpreting white blood cell counts of lithium-treated patients with infections and other conditions requiring leukocyte count monitoring.

Geriatric. Since the glomerular filtration rate decreases with age, smaller doses of lithium may be required to reach therapeutic levels. Additionally, the increased number of physical disorders among elderly patients stresses the importance of pretreatment evaluation and careful monitoring during therapy, especially because these patients are often under dietary restriction and receiving other medications.

Although any patient may experience side effects at toxic lithium levels, older patients may delevop serious adverse reaction at therapeutic levels. Smith and Helms (1982) found a greater incidence of moderate to severe adverse effects among lithium-treated patients age sixty-five and over compared to a younger group. Most prominent were symptoms of neurotoxicity. The authors noted that moderate to severe reactions occured mainly in elderly patients with levels between 1.2 and 1.5 mEq/L and concluded that 1.2 mEq/L should be the upper limit of therapeutic range in geriatric patients (Smith & Helms, 1982).

Pregnancy and Breast Feeding. Pregnancy in a lithium-treated patient raises a number of considerations. During pregnancy, lithium clearance increases 10 to 100 percent, returning to normal at delivery. Any compensatory increase in dosage should be monitored frequently during pregnancy and then reduced shortly before delivery to avoid toxicity (Reisberg & Gerson, 1979). If sodium restriction is necessary, dosage should be reduced or toxicity may ensue.

Lithium does cross the placental barrier, and a number of cardiac malformations, particularly Ebstein's anomaly (tricuspid valve malformation), have been discovered at higher than expected rates in newborns exposed to lithium *in utero*. Lithium treatment should be avoided during pregnancy, at least during the first trimester (Goldberg & DiMascio, 1978). Of course, the risk of a major affective episode may outweigh the teratogenic risks. Since animal data indicate an increase in teratogenic effects with high peaks in lithium serum concentration, individual doses should be small and frequent (Weinstein & Goldfield, 1975). Sustained-release preparations may be of special value in avoiding plasma peaks.

The issue of breast feeding also is clouded. Breast milk concentration of lithium is about half that in the nursing mother's serum. Because an infant's regulatory and excretory functions are not well developed, one point of view holds that breast feeding by a mother receiving lithium should be avoided. Conversely, a few months exposure to lower lithium plasma concentrations (about one-third of the mothers after the first week of life) than were experienced *in utero* probably represents little risk and may well be outweighed by the psychological, nutritional, and immunologic benefits of breast feeding (Linden & Rich, 1983).

Drug-Drug Interactions.   Because lithium's kinetics are closely tied to fluid and sodium balance, the concurrent use of diuretics is of concern. Thiazide diuretics cause an increase in serum lithium levels, probably by blocking sodium resorption in the proximal tubule, allowing selective retention of lithium. Toxicity is an obvious risk, but the combination can be used safely with close monitoring of lithium levels and appropriate dosage adjustment. Once stable, levels are consistent. Similar caution probably should be taken with potassium-sparing diuretics. Although a single dose of spironolactone appears to decrease lithium levels, administration over several days causes a consistent rise in serum lithium despite little change in external lithium balance (Gualtieri & Powell, 1978; Solomon, 1978).

Other diuretics tend to lower serum lithium levels, risking a psychiatric relapse. Acetazolamide (carbonic anhydrase inhibitor) and mannitol (osmotic diuretic) cause a large increase in lithium excretion and have been used in treatment of lithium intoxication (Jefferson, Greist, & Baudhuin, 1981).

Jefferson and Kalin (1979) administered furosemide over a 2-week period to lithium-treated individuals and found no significant change in serum lithium, whereas hydrochlorothiazide increased levels in the same subjects. The authors suggested that substantial amounts of lithium may be reabsorbed in the loop of Henle, requiring no modification of lithium dosage when used with a loop diuretic (furosemide, ethacrynic acid).

Nonsteroidal anti-inflammatory drugs (NSAID) may cause decreased elimination of lithium (Ragheb, et al., 1980). Indomethacin in doses of 150 mg daily can suppress lithium clearance by 30%, perhaps by inhibiting prostaglandin-dependent mechanisms in the distal tubule (Frolich et al., 1979). Ibuprofen may have a similar effect (Kilbourne, Keewhan, Jones, Thacker, & Field Investigation Team, 1982). Although the status of other NSAID remains unclarified, all of these agents should be used cautiously in conjunction with lithium. Animal data suggest that steroids may increase the excretion of lithium. Adverse interactions in humans have not been established, and lithium has been used to prevent steroid-induced hypomania (Jefferson, Greist, & Baudhuin, 1981).

Diuretics are often used in patients with cardiovascular disease, and lithium may interact unfavorably with at least two other cardiac medications. A few case reports have associated the antihypertensive methyldopa with neurotoxic symptoms in lithium-treated patients, although the drugs also have been used together without problems (Sandifer, 1978). Lithium also has been cited as potentiating digitalis-induced arrhythmias, possibly by depleting intracellular potassium. This interaction is probably rare, and the combination is considered safe.

Since lithium has an antithyroid effect, it is not surprising that other antithyroids, iodine, and the thioamides (propylthiouracil, methimazole, carbimazole, and methylthiouracil) may have an additive or synergistic effect when used with lithium. Such combinations have been used in treating thyrotoxicosis.

Neuromuscular blocking agents should be used cautiously in lithium-treated patients. Animal data and a few case reports suggest that lithium may prolong the effects of succinylcholine and pancuronium bromide (Jefferson, Greist, & Baudhuin, 1981). As such, lithium-treated patients probably should have the medication discontinued, when possible, prior to surgery or ECT. In fact, the combination of lithium therapy and ECT has been associated with aggravation of post-ECT confusion (Small, Kellams, Milstein, & Small, 1980). The combination of lithium and haloperidol also has been associated with mental clouding and even coma, tremor, and seizures. That the haloperidol lithium combination has synergistic adverse effects is unsettled, but it would seem wise to avoid using high doses of these medications together (Tupin & Schuller, 1978).

ANTIANXIETY DRUGS

Whether triggered by internal or external stimuli, anxiety, with its pervasive quality of apprehension and multiple somatic symptoms, is a frequent patient complaint. Not surprisingly, antianxiety agents are widely prescribed both to outpatients and hospitalized patients (Greenblatt & Shader, 1974). Since a number of disease states (peptic ulcer, inflammatory bowel disease, epilepsy, bronchial asthma, hypertension, ischemic heart disease, for example) can be aggravated by anxiety, the use of anxiolytics in physically ill patients can be of considerable benefit.

The barbiturates and meprobamate were once extremely popular drugs for the treatment of anxiety. However, tolerance and physical dependence proved to be major problems and potential suicide use a high risk. Antidepressants, especially those with sedating properties (amitriptyline, doxepin), antihistaminics (hydroxyzine, diphenhydramine), and antipsychotics (thioridazine) also have been used as antianxiety agents, but all three groups are strongly anticholinergic, and their anxiolytic actions are weaker than those of meprobamate and the barbiturates. Moreover, the antidepressants and antipsychotics are associated with a number of serious side effects, and tricyclic antidepressants are particularly dangerous in overdosage (Hollister, 1978).

Benzodiazepines are now the dominant group of antianxiety drugs. Overall, they are more effective anxiolytics than other available drugs and appear to be one of the safest classes of drugs ever introduced. Although physical dependence and withdrawal may occur, these drugs otherwise are associated with few serious adverse reactions, and suicide potential is essentially nonexistent. Moreover, the benzodiazepines are less likely to induce metabolizing enzymes than are the barbiturates or meprobamate (Finkle, McCloskey, & Goodman, 1979; Hollister, 1981a).

Although the mechanism of action of benzodiazepines is not completely understood, most data suggest that they increase the activity of gamma-aminobutyric acid (GABA), a central neurotransmitter with inhibitory actions. Some evidence suggests that benzodiazepines bind at specific benzodiazepine receptors that may be closely associated with GABA binding and activity (Snyder, 1981).

The major indication for benzodiazepine treatment is significant anxiety, including anticipatory, situational, traumatic, and free-floating anxiety states. Usually these conditions are self-limited or episodic, and most authorities suggest that benzodiazepines be used for brief periods only (Edwards and Mendlincott, 1980), although others suggest that the occasional patient with chronic anxiety may benefit from long-term use with few complications (Hollister, Conley, Britt, & Shur, 1981). Panic states and phobic anxiety appear to respond better to TCA or MAOI, although alprazolam, a newly released benzodiazepine, seems to be quite effective in these disorders.

Benzodiazepines also are used as muscle relaxants, hypnotics, anesthetics (for endoscopy procedures, cardioversion, and labor and delivery), and premedication before general anesthesia. They also are used to control status epilepticus and to suppress symptoms of alcohol withdrawal. Since they suppress slow-wave sleep, benzodiazepines can control night terrors, enuresis, and somnambulism (Greenblatt & Shader, 1974; Hollister, 1978).

Benzodiazepines can be pharmacokinetically divided into the long-acting compounds (chlordiazepoxide, diazepam, prazepam chlorazepate, and flurazepam) and the short-to-intermediate agents (oxazepam, lorazepam, and alprazolam). Generally, the long-acting drugs undergo oxidative biotransformation into a number of metabolites, some active, whereas the short-acting drugs are conjugated and have no important active metabolites. Accumulation can be extensive with long-acting benzodiazepines and elimination slow. Protein binding is high in both groups (Greenblatt & Shader, 1980; Hollister, 1981a).

Chlordiazepoxide is well absorbed orally but slowly and erratically absorbed after intramuscular administration. The parent drug is metabolized to several active metabolites, and elimination half-life is 8 to 48 h. Similarly, diazepam is rapidly and completely absorbed when given orally, but intramuscular dosages produce lower plasma levels than does oral administration. Diazepam attains highest plasma concentrations when given intravenously for treatment of status epilepticus or alcohol withdrawal and as an anesthetic or surgical premedication (Hollister, 1978, 1981). Prazepam is actually a drug precursor, since it is rapidly converted by the liver to N-desmethyldiazepam. Chlorazepate acts similarly, undergoing hydroxylation and decarboxylation in gastric acid, appearing in the systemic circulation as N-desmethyldiazepam. The half-life of this metabolite is 30 to 96 h. Flurazepam also can be considered a drug precursor, since it is rapidly converted to desalkylflurazepam, a long-acting metabolite with a half-life of 50 to 100 h (Hollister, 1978; Tedeschi et al., 1958). Although flurazepam is marketed as a hypnotic, it is probably no more effective as a hypnotic than any other benzodiazepine (Hollister, 1978).

The short-acting benzodiazepines oxazepam (half-life 7 to 20 h) and lorazepam (half-life 10 to 20 h) undergo simple conjugation and produce no active metabolites. Steady-state kinetics are reached more quickly than with the long-acting benzodiazepines, and cumulative effects are unlikely. However, more frequent dosing is required for maintenance, and abrupt discontinuation is more apt to produce uncomfortable symptoms (Hollister, 1981a). Lorazepam given by intramuscular injection is well absorbed, an advantage over diazepam and chlordiazepoxide. Diazepam given intravenously tends to lose its therapeutic effects quickly because of rapid and extensive tissue distribution. Lorazepam has a longer duration of action (sedative, amnestic, and anticonvulsive effects) than diazepam when given intravenously (Greenblatt & Shader, 1978).

Alprazolam, a recently introduced triazolobenzodiazepine, appears to have a half-life of about 12 h. Its metabolism and the nature of its metabolites are not completely understood. The drug shows great promise for the treatment of phobic anxiety and panic states and perhaps mixed anxiety-depression states.

Side Effects

Neurological.   Sedation is the most frequent side effect of benzodiazepines. Because of their cumulative effects, the longer-acting agents may produce considerable dulling of cognition and impairment of motor skills (Greenblatt & Shader, 1974; Zisook & DeVaul, 1977).

Physical dependence may develop during prolonged treatment with substantial doses of benzodiazepines. Abrupt discontinuation can lead to a severe withdrawal syndrome, including seizures. Onset is earlier and intensity more severe with lorazepam and oxazepam; plasma elimination is more gradual for the long-acting agents (Hollister, 1981a).

Benzodiazepine action at both brainstem and spinal cord levels produces skeletal muscle relaxation, and these drugs are often used to relieve spasm associated with a number of neurological disorders. High doses usually are required, and best results are obtained with continuous intravenous administration (Greenblatt & Shader, 1974).

Cardiovascular.   The benzodiazepines appear to be relatively free of major cardiovascular side effects. Even large amounts of orally ingested drug fail to produce any significant hypotension, reduction in myocardial performance, or arrhythmias. Hypotension has been observed with intravenous diazepam given to debilitated patients pretreated with other centrally acting depressants. Benzodiazepine injection can cause local irritation, phlebitis, and venous thrombosis (Hollister, 1978).

No serious contraindication exists for the oral or intramuscular administration of benzodiazepines to patients with cardiovascular disease. In fact, fairly liberal use of benzodiazepines following myocardial infarction correlates with a decrease in cardiovascular morbidity and mortality (Freebury, Brown, Moldofsky, & Howley, 1978).

Respiratory.   Any centrally acting depressant, including the benzodiazepines, may precipitate acute respiratory acidosis in patients with respiratory disease by decreasing ventilatory effort. Apnea can occur when diazepam or lorazepam are given intravenously, especially in debilitated patients or those who have received other depressant drugs (Van Praag, 1978). Modest doses of chlordiazepoxide can cause a rise in venous carbon dioxide tension and attenuate forced expiratory volume (Hollister, 1978). Additionally, if a patient's complaints of insomnia can be explained by sleep apnea, any hypnotic medication should be avoided, since the risk of further respiratory depression or sudden death are very real (Mendelson, Garnett, & Gillin, 1981).

Gastrointestinal.   Infrequently, a number of nonspecific, minor gastrointestinal disturbances have been associated with benzodiazepine treatment. Assuming there is no major interference with absorption, antianxiety drugs may well benefit patients with gastrointestinal disorders aggravated by substantial anxiety. Patients with reduced gastric acid may not be able to utilize chlorazepate.

Hepatic.   Chlordiazepoxide, diazepam, and flurazepam have been associated with cholestatic jaundice in case reports (Reynolds, Lloyd, & Slinger, 1981), usually confounded by the use of other medications. Considering the wide use of benzodiazepines, the frequency of hepatotoxic reactions seems exceedingly low.

In patients with preexisting liver disease the elimination half-life of chlordiazepoxide, diazepam, and desmethyldiazepam are markedly increased, whereas the pharmacokinetics of lorazepam and oxazepam show little change. Thus, the short-acting agents may be preferable in patients with hepatic dysfunction. Any sedating drug should be used cautiously in patients with cirrhosis to diminish the risk of precipitating encephalopathy (Hoyumpa, 1978).

Renal. The benzodiazepines do not appear to have any significant effect on renal function. However, patients with renal failure and electrolyte disturbances should be considered sensitive to sedative effects. The elimination of active metabolites of chlordiazepoxide is in part accomplished through the kidneys, and the drug probably should be avoided in renal failure. Strain (1975) has suggested that diazepam is the drug of choice in patients with renal compromise, since diazepam is fully metabolized through the liver and no dosage reduction is required. Since the short-acting agents are metabolized to inactive glucuronides, they would seem to be similarly useful.

Metabolic/Endocrine. In the presence of significantly lowered albumin levels, the risk of oversedation from diazepam increases, probably through reduced protein binding of active drug (Greenblatt & Shader, 1974; Hollister, 1978). Such an effect would be expected with other benzodiazepines. Although it is important to distinguish anxiety and depression from disorders of thyroid metabolism (Devaris & Mehlman, 1979), there is little consistent evidence that benzodiazepines interfere with laboratory evaluation of thyroid function. However, diazepam can interfere with the 1.0-mg dexamethasone suppression test used in the diagnosis of major depression and Cushing's disease (Carroll et al., 1981).

Hematalogic. Rare case reports have associated benzodiazepines with blood dyscrasias, but cause and effect are difficult to determine (Finkle et al., 1979).

Geriatric. Because cytochrome P450 oxidase decreases with age, the plasma half-life of long-acting benzodiazepines increases considerably with age, and cumulative effects can be pronounced. The half-life of lorazepam and oxazepam does not increase significantly with age, and these agents seem preferable for geriatric patients (Hoyumpa, 1978).

Pregnancy and Breast Feeding. When used early in pregnancy, benzodiazepines have been associated with an increase incidence of cleft lip and cleft palate. The risk appears to be low, but it would be wise to avoid benzodiazepine treatment during the first trimester of pregnancy, especially if the expectant parents have a family history of such deformities. High doses of benzodiazepines late in pregnancy may cause neonatal jaundice, hypotonia, and respiratory depression (Greenblatt & Shader, 1974). Benzodiazepines do appear in human milk, but nursing seems to present little risk to the newborn (Ananth, 1978).

Drug-Drug Interactions. In part, the efficacy and low frequency of side effects of benzodiazepines have promoted the clinical popularity of these medications. Similarly, the benzodiazepines are associated with relatively few unfavorable interactions with other medications, especially in contrast to the barbiturates. However, some important considerations of pharmacologic interactions do exist.

Sedation is the prominent side effect of benzodiazepines. Generally, administration of benzodiazepines with any other drugs with sedative properties (antidepressants, antipsychotics, anticonvulsants, and the like) enhances the risk of oversedation. Alcohol presents a similar risk, as do over-the-counter "sleep aids" and antihistamines. Stimulants such as amphetamines and large amounts of caffeine can be expected to interfere with the antianxiety effects of benzodiazepines. Similarly, the benzodiazepines have been reported to increase amphetamine-induced hyperactivity and stereotypy.

Benzodiazepines do possess anticonvulsant properties. However, diazepam and chlordiazepoxide may increase phenytoin metabolism. Also, anticonvulsants may increase metabolism and clearance of benzodiazepines. Conversely, disulfiram may decrease clearance of chlordiazepoxide (Gualtieri & Powell, 1978).

Alcohol appears to delay diazepam absorption, although absorption is still complete. Benzodiazepine absorption can also be hindered by antacids. Cimetidine, the histamine-2 receptor blocker, also is used to decrease gastric acidity. Cimetidine appears to inhibit cytochrome P450 oxidase, interfering with metabolism and raising serum levels of diazepam, chlordiazepoxide, and perhaps other long-acting benzodiazepines (Ruffalo, Thompson, & Segel, 1981). Since oxazepam and lorazepam are not oxidatively metabolized, they are not affected by this interaction. Animal data indicate that estrogens also may suppress cytochrome P450, and chronic use of low-dose estrogen-containing oral contraceptives has been shown to decrease diazepam elimination (Abernathy et al., 1982). A similar effect might be expected with other long-acting benzodiazepines, whereas lorazepam and oxazepam may offer a particular advantage.

REFERENCES

Abernathy, D. R., Greenblatt, D. J., Divoli, M., Arendt, R., Ochs, H. R., & Shader, R. I. (1982). Impairment of diazepam metabolism by low-dose estrogen containing oral-contraceptive steroids. *New England Journal of Medicine, 306,* 791–792.

Albertini, R. S., & Penders, T. M. (1978). Agranulocytosis associated with tricyclics. *Journal of Clinical Psychiatry, 39,* 483–485.

Ananth, J. (1978). Side effects from psychotropic agents excreted through breast feeding. *American Journal of Psychiatry, 135,* 801–805.

Annitto, W., Prien, R., & Gershon, S. (1980). The lithium ion: Is it specific for mania? In R. H. Belmake & H. M. van Praag (Eds.), *Mania: An evolving concept.* (pp. 127–142) New York: Spectrum.

Bennett, W. M., Singer, I., & Coggins, C. H. (1970). A practical guide to drug usage in adult patients with impaired renal function. *Journal of the American Medical Association, 214,* 1468–1475.

Bernstein, J. G. (1978). Medical-psychiatric drug interactions. In T. P. Hackett & N. H. Cassem (Eds.), *MGH handbook of general hospital psychiatry.* St. Louis: C. V. Mosby.

Bernstein, J. G. (1979). Antipsychotic drugs in the general hospital: Uses and cautions. *Psychosomatics, 20,* 335, 339, 342–343.

Bigger, J. T., Kantor, S. J., Glassman, A. H., & Perel, J. M. (1978). Cardiovascular effects of tricyclic antidepressant drugs. In M. A. Lipton, A. Di Mascio, & K. F. Killam (Eds.), *Psychopharmacology: A generation of progress.* (pp. 1033–1046) New York: Raven Press.

Blackwell, B. (1981). Adverse effects of antidepressant drugs: Part 1. Monoamine oxidase inhibitors and tricyclics. *Drugs, 21,* 201–219.

Carroll, J. B., Feinberg, M., Greden, J. F., Tarika, J., Albala, A. A., Haskett, R. F., James, N., Kronfol, Z., Lohr, N., Steiner, M., DeVigne, J. P., & Young, E. (1981). A specific laboratory test for the diagnosis of melancholia. *Archives of General Psychiatry, 38,* 15–22.

Charalampous, K. D., & Keepers, G. A. (1978). Major side effects of antipsychotic drugs. *Journal of Family Practice, 6,* 993–1001.

Clark, R. W., Schmidt, H. S., Schaal, S. F., Boudoulas, H., & Schuller, D. (1979). Sleep apnea: Treatment with protriptyline. *Neurology, 29,* 1287–1292.

Cooper, D. S., Gelenberg, A. J., Wojcik, J. C., Saxe, V. C., Ridgeway, E. C., & Maloof, F. (1981). The effect of amoxapine and imipramine on serum prolactin levels. *Archives of Internal Medicine, 141,* 1023–1025.

Cooper, T. B., Simpson, G. M., Lee, J. H., & Bergner, P. E. (1978). Evaluation of a slow release lithium carbonate formulation. *American Journal of Psychiatry, 135,* 917–922.

Dahl, S. G. (1982). Active metabolites of neuroleptic drugs: Possible contribution to therapeutic and toxic effects. *Therapeutic Drug Monitor, 4,* 33–40.

Davidson, J., & Wenger, T. (1982). Using antidepressants in patients with cardiovascular disease. *Drug Therapy, 12,* 55–64.

Demers, R. G., & Henniger, G. R. (1971). Electrocardiographic T-wave changes during lithium carbonate treatment. *Journal of the American Medical Association, 218,* 381–386.

Demers, R.G., Lukesh, R., & Prichard, J. (1970). Convulsions during lithium therapy. *Lancet, 2,* 315–316.

Devaris, D. P., & Mehlman, I. (1979). Psychiatric presentations of endocrine and metabolic disorders. *Primary Care, 6,* 245–265.

Ducomb, L., & Baldessarini, R. J. (1977). Timing and risk of bone marrow depression by psychotropic drugs. *American Journal of Psychiatry, 134,* 1294–1295.

Edwards, R. A., & Medlincott, R. W. (1980). Advantages and disadvantages of benzodiazepine prescription. *New Zealand Medical Journal, 92,* 357–359.

Finkle, B. S., McCloskey, K. L., & Goodman, L. S. (1979). Diazepam and drug associated deaths: A survey in the United States and Canada. *Journal of the American Medical Association, 242,* 429–434.

Flaherty, J. A., & Lahmeyer, H. W. (1978). Laryngeal-pharyngeal dystonia as a possible cause of asphyxia with haloperidol treatment. *American Journal of Psychiatry, 135,* 1414–1415.

Franks, R. D., Dubovsky, S. L., Lifshitz, M., Coen, P., Subryan, V., & Walker, S. (1982). Long term lithium carbonate therapy causes hyperparathyroidism. *Archives of General Psychiatry, 39,* 1074–1077.

Freebury, D. R., Brown, G. M., Moldofsky, H., & Howley, T. (1978). Growth hormone and cortisol responses, tranquilizer usage, and their association with survival from myocardial infarction. *Psychosomatic Medicine, 40,* 462–477.

Frolich, J. C., Leftwich, R., Ragheb, M., Dates, J. A., Reimann, I., & Buchanan, D. (1979). Indomethacin increases plasma lithium. *British Medical Journal, 1,* 1115–1116.

Gershon, S., & Yuwiler, A. (1960). Lithium ion: A specific psychopharmacological approach to the treatment of mania. *Journal of Neuropsychiatry, 1,* 229–241.

Ghadirian, A. M., & Lehman, H. E. (1980). Neurological side effects of lithium: Organic brain syndrome, seizures, extrapyramidal side effects and EEG changes. *Comprehensive Psychiatry, 21,* 327–335.

Goldberg, H. L., & DiMascio, A. (1978). Psychotropic drugs in pregnancy. In M. A. Lipton, A. DiMascio, & K. F. Killam (Eds.), *Psychopharmacology: A generation of progress.* (pp. 1047–1055) New York: Raven Press.

Gramm, L. F., Pederson, O. L., Kristensen, C. B., & Kraugh-Sorensen, P. (1982). Drug level monitoring in psychoparmacology: Usefulness and clinical problems, with special references to tricyclic antidepressants. *Therapeutic Drug Monitor, 4,* 17–25.

Granacher, R. P., & Baldessarini, R. J. (1975). Physostigmine: Its use in acute anticholinergic syndrome with antidepressant and antiparkinson drugs. *Archives of General Psychiatry, 32,* 375–380.

Greenblatt, D. J., Gross, P. L., Harris, J., Shader, R., & Circaulo, D. (1978). Fatal hyperthermia following haloperidol therapy of sedative hypnotic withdrawal. *Journal of Clinical Psychiatry, 39,* 673–675.

Greenblatt, D. J., & Shader, R. I. (1974). Benzodiazepines. *New England Journal of Medicine, 291,* 1011–1015, 1239–1243.

Greenblatt, D. J., & Shader, R. I. (1978). Prazepam and clorazepam, two new benzodiazepines. *New England Journal of Medicine, 299,* 1342–1344.

Greenblatt, D. J., & Shader, R. I. (1980). Pharmacokinetic aspects of anxiolytic drug therapy. *Canadian Journal of Neurological Science, 7,* 269–270.

Gualtieri, C. T., & Powell, S. F. (1978). Psychoactive drug interactions. *Journal of Clinical Psychiatry, 39,* 720–729.

Hayes, J. R., Born, G. F., & Rosenbaum, A. H. (1977). Incidence of orthostatic hypotension in patients with primary affective disorders treated with tricyclic antidepressants. *Mayo Clinic Proceedings, 52,* 509–512.

Hollister, L. E. (1964). Adverse reactions to phenothiazines. *Journal of the American Medical Association, 189,* 311–313.

Hollister, L. E. (1978). *Clinical pharmacology of psychotherapeutic drugs.* New York: Churchill Livingstone.

Hollister, L. E. (1981a). Pharmacology and pharmacokinetics of the minor tranquilizers. *Psychiatric Annals, 11* (Suppl), 26–31.

Hollister, L. E. (1981b). "Second generation" antidepressant drugs. *Psychosomatics, 22,* 872–879.

Hollister, L. E., Conley, F. K., Britt, R. H., & Shur, L. (1981). Long term use of diazepam. *Journal of the American Medical Association, 246,* 1568–1570.

Hoyumpa, A. (1978). Disposition and elimination of minor tranquilizers in the aged and in patients with liver disease. *Southern Medical Journal, 71,* 23–28.

Jagdish, C. M., & Pereira, M. (1982). Tricyclic antidepressants in the treatment of peptic ulcer disease. *Archives of Internal Medicine, 142,* 273–275.

Jamm, M. W., & Bitar, A. H. (1982). Respiratory dyskinesia. *Psychosomatics, 23,* 764–765.

Jefferson, J. W. (1975). A review of the cardiovascular effects and toxicity of tricyclic antidepressants. *Psychosomatic Medicine, 37,* 160–179.

Jefferson, J. W., Greist, J. H., & Baudhuin, M. (1981). Lithium: Interactions with other drugs. *Journal of Clinical Psychopharmacology, 1,* 124–134.

Jefferson, J. W., & Kalin, N. H. (1979). Serum lithium levels and long term diuretic use. *Journal of the American Medical Association, 241,* 1134–1136.

Kane, J., Rifkin, A., Quitkin, F., & Klein, D. F. (1978). Extrapyramidal side effects with lithium treatment. *American Journal of Psychiatry, 135,* 851–853.

Kilbourne, E. M., Keewhan, C., Jones, T. S., Thacker, S. B., & Field Investigation Team (1982). Risk factors for heatstroke: A case control study. *Journal of the American Medical Association, 247,* 3332–3336.

Klein, D. F., Zitrin, C. M., & Woerner, M. (1978). Antidepressants, anxiety, panic, and phobia. In M. A. Lipton, A. DiMascio, & K. F. Killam (Eds.), *Psychopharmacology: A generation of progress.* (pp. 1401–1410) New York: Raven Press.

Levenson, A. J., Beard, O. W., & Murphy, M. L. (1980). Major tranquilizers and heart disease: To use or not to use. *Geriatrics, 35,* 55–61.

Liebowitz, M. R., Quitkin, F. M., Stewart, J. W., McGrath, P. J., Harrison, W., Schwartz, D., Rabkin, J., Tricamo, E., & Klein, D. F. (1981). Phenelzine and imipramine in atypical depression. *Psychopharmacology Bulletin, 17,* 159–161.

Linden, S., & Rich, C. L. (1983). The use of lithium during pregnancy and lactation. *Journal of Clinical Psychiatry, 44,* 358–361.

Lundborg, P., & Engel, J. (1978). Neurochemical brain changes associated with behavioral disturbances after early treatment with psychotropic drugs. In A. Vernadakis, E. Giacobini, & G. Filogamo (Eds.), *Maturation of neurotransmission.* (pp. 226–235) Basel: S. Karger.

Mendelson, W. B., Garnett, D., & Gillin, J. C. (1981). Flurazepam-induced sleep apnea syndrome in a patient with insomnia and mild sleep related respiratory changes. *Journal of Nervous and Mental Disorders, 169,* 261–264.

Mitchell, J. E., & Mackenzie, T. B. (1982). Cardiac effects of lithium therapy in man: A review. *Journal of Clinical Psychiatry, 43,* 47–51.

Muller, O. F., Goodman, N., & Bellet, S. (1961). The hypotensive effect of imipramine hydrochloride in patients with cardiovascular disease. *Clinical Pharmacology and Therapeutics, 2,* 300–307.

Murburg, M., Anton, R. F., Nelson J. C., & Atlow, P. I. (1982). Noninvasive measurement of cardiac ejection fraction during desipramine treatment. *Psychosomatics, 23,* 759–761.

Nasrallah, H. (1978). Factors in influencing phenothiazine-induced ECG changes. *American Journal of Psychiatry, 135,* 118–119.

Neil, J. F., Himmelhoch, J. M., & Licata, S. M. (1976). Emergence of myasthenia gravis during treatment with lithium carbonate. *Archives of General Psychiatry, 33,* 1090–1092.

Neshkes, R. E., & Jarvik, L. F. (1982). Clinical psychiatry and cardiovascular disease in the elderly. *Psychiatric Clinics of North America, 5,* 171–179.

Ragheb, M., Ban, T. A., Buchanan, D., & Frolich, J. C. (1980). Interaction of indomethacin and ibuprofen with lithium in manic patients under a steady-state lithium level. *Journal of Clinical Psychiatry, 41,* 397–398.

Ramsey, T. A., & Cox, M. (1982). Lithium and the kidney: A review. *American Journal of Psychiatry, 139,* 443–449.

Raskind, M. A., Vieth, R. C., Barnes, R., & Gumbrecht, G. (1982). Cardiovascular and antidepressant effects of imipramine in the treatment of secondary depression in patients with ischemic heart disease. *American Journal of Psychiatry, 139,* 1114–1117.

Regestein, Q. R., Reich, P., & Mufson, M. J. (1983). Narcolepsy: An initial clinical approach. *Journal of Clinical Psychiatry, 44,* 166–172.

Reisberg, B., & Gershon, S. (1979). Side effects associated with lithium therapy. *Archives of General Psychiatry, 36,* 879–887.

Remick, R. A., & Fine, S. H. (1979). Antipsychotic drugs and seizures. *Journal of Clinical Psychiatry, 40,* 78–80.

Reynolds, R., Lloyd, D. A., & Slinger, R. P. (1981). Cholestatic jaundice induced by flurazepam hydrochloride. *Canadian Medical Association Journal, 124,* 893–894.

Rikfin, A., Saraf, K., Kane, J., Ross, D., & Klein, D. F. (1980). A comparison of trimipramine and imipramine: A controlled study. *Journal of Clinical Psychiatry, 41,* 124–129.

Risch, S. C., & Janowsky, D. S. (1981). Trazodone. *Psychiatric Annals, 11,* 396–400.

Robinson, D. S., & Barker, E. (1976). Tricyclic antidepressant cardiotoxicity. *Journal of the American Medical Association, 236,* 2089–2090.

Ruffalo, R. L., Thompson, J. F., & Segel, J. L. (1981). Diazepam-cimetidine drug interaction: A clinically significant effect. *Southern Medical Journal, 74,* 1075–1078.

Salzman, C. (1982). Key concepts in geriatric psychopharmacology: Altered pharmacokinetics and polypharmacy. *Psychiatric Clinics of North America, 5,* 181–189.

Sandifer, M. G. (1978). The hypertensive psychiatric patient: Pharmacologic problems. *Journal of Clinical Psychiatry, 39,* 700–702.

Schwartz, B. (1978). Current concepts in ophthalmology: The glaucomas. *New England Journal of Medicine, 299,* 182–184.

Singer, I., & Rotenberg, D. (1973). Mechanisms of lithium action. *New England Journal of Medicine, 289,* 254–260.

Siris, S. G., & Rifkin, A. (1981). The problem of psychopharmacotherapy in the medically ill. *Psychiatric Clinics of North America, 4,* 379–390.

Small, J. G., Kellams, J. J., Milstein, V., & Small, I. F. (1980). Complications of electroconvulsive treatment combined with lithium. *Biological Psychiatry, 15,* 103–112.

Smego, R. A., & Durack, D. T. (1982). The neuroleptic malignant syndrome. *Archives of Internal Medicine, 142,* 1183–1185.

Smith, R. E., & Helms, P.M. (1982). Adverse effects of lithium therapy in the acutely ill elderly patient. *Journal of Clinical Psychiatry, 43,* 94–99.

Snyder, S. H. (1981). Opiate and benzodiazepine receptors. *Psychosomatics, 22,* 986–989.

Solomon, K. (1978). Combined use of lithium and diuretics. *Southern Medical Journal, 71,* 1098–1104.

Strain, J. J. (1975). Psychopharmacological treatment of the medically ill. In J. Strain & S. Grossman (Eds.), *Psychological care of the medically ill: A primer in liaison psychiatry.* (pp. 108-122) New York: Appleton-Century-Crofts.

Tedeschi, D. H., Benigni, J. P., Elder, C., Yeager, J. C., & Flanigan, J. V. (1958). Effects of various phenothiazines on minimal electroshock seizure threshold and spontaneous motor activity of mice. *Journal of Pharmacology and Experimental Therapeutics, 123,* 35–38.

Tilkian, A. G., Schroeder, J. S., Kao, J., & Hultgren, H. (1976). Effect of lithium on cardiovascular performance: Report on extended ambulatory monitoring and exercise testing before and during lithium therapy. *American Journal of Cardiology, 38,* 701–708.

Tupin, J. P., & Schuller, A. B. (1978). Lithium and haloperidol incompatibility reviewed. *Psychiatric Journal of the University of Ottawa, 4,* 245–251.

Van Praag, H. M. (1978). *Psychotropic drugs: A guide for the practitioner.* New York: Brunner/Mazel.

Vieth, R. C., Raskind, M. A., Caldwell, J. H., Barnes, R. F., Gumbrecht, G., & Ritchie, J. L. (1982). Cardiovascular effects of tricyclic antidepressants in depressed patients with chronic heart disease. *New England Journal of Medicine, 306,* 954–959.

Weinstein, M. R., & Goldfield, M. D. (1975). Administration of lithium during pregnancy. In F. N. Johnson, (Ed.), *Lithium: Research and therapy.* (pp. 237–264) London: Academic Press.

Zavodnick, S. (1978). A pharmacological and theoretical comparison of high and low potency neuroleptics. *Journal of Clinical Psychiatry, 39,* 332–336.

Zetin, M., Plon, L., Nosratola, V., Cramer, M., & Greco, D. (1981). Lithium carbonate dose and serum level relationships in chronic hemodialysis patients. *American Journal of Psychiatry, 138,* 1387–1388.

Zisook, S., & Devaul, R. A. (1977). Adverse behavioral effects of benzodiazepines. *Journal of Family Practice, 5,* 963–966.

Chapter 4

PATIENTS WITH PAIN

Timothy Bayer

Pain is a complicated phenomenon. It cannot be understood or treated adequately without consideration of many different factors. Early in their training most physicians encounter patients who complain bitterly of pain but in whom no lesion can be demonstrated. Other patients have pain that persists far beyond the time most physicians expect it to last. Beecher's (1959) classic study of the pain associated with war injuries showed that there is often little relationship between the extent of the injury, the amount of reported pain, and the desire for relief of the pain through the use of narcotics. Some of his injured patients required very little pain control. He concluded that this was related in part to the meaning of the wound, providing a socially acceptable reason for returning home from the war. Thus, pain is a phenomenon that is influenced and determined on many levels, all of which interact with each other. It is very difficult for physicians to understand and treat patients who complain of pain, without some knowledge of the biological, psychological, and social determinants of pain and pain complaints. Engel's biopsychosocial model (1977) is therefore generally useful, but a more specific model is desirable.

In the past 15 years there has been a marked increase in the number of experimental and theoretical discussions of the problem of pain. It is still not possible to integrate fully the contributions of each of the various models available for dealing with pain, but it is useful to have some knowledge of what each model contributes to both the evaluation and the treatment of pain.

The importance of these various ways of understanding pain varies. One of the most important concepts recently developed is the distinction between acute and chronic pain. There is clearly an important distinction in terms of the biological function of pain in the two conditions. There are also important differences in their clinical presentation and available treatment methods. The importance of psychological and social factors also differs in acute and chronic pain; they are particularly important in dealing with patients with chronic pain. Sternbach (1981) has noted that in chronic pain the pain has become overdetermined by psychological as well as by somatic forces. He argues that in such cases the pain is no longer a symptom of the disease but has become the disease itself.

Difficulties in discussing the problem of pain arise even at the basic level of consensus on definition. To say that pain is whatever the patient says it is may eliminate the problem of definition, but it is not necessarily useful, particularly in deciding on treatment. As an abstract concept pain can be discussed on many levels. In an attempt to standardize the discussion, the International Association for the Study of Pain (1979) has defined pain as "an unpleasant sensory and emotional experience associated with actual or potential tissue damage or described in terms of such damage."

BIOLOGICAL CONSIDERATIONS

The study of the biology of pain has been marked by several recent advances in our understanding of the biological mechanisms involved in the processing of pain by the nervous system. Of particular recent interest are the findings regarding the neuroregulators and neurotransmitters involved in the transmission and processing of pain-induced impulses.

At the level of the pain receptors much attention has been paid to what are called algesic substances. These substances produce pain when injected into tissue and are thought to act as chemical mediators on the sensory nerve ending. They include serotonin, histamine, and bradykinin (Terenius, 1981). Prostaglandins have not been shown to have a direct effect in producing impulses from the sensory nerve endings but do potentiate or sensitize the nociceptor (Terenius, 1981). Aspirin and other medications inhibit the synthesis of prostaglandins and thus act to decrease the sensitivity of the pain receptors. In experimental pain, there tends to be a good correlation between the amount of discharge from the sensory neuron and the subjectively reported level of pain (Zimmerman, 1981).

The sensitivity of the nociceptors also is influenced by smooth muscle tone and by sympathetic discharge. This sympathetic influence on the excitability of the nociceptors may lead to some types of chronic pain. This occurs particularly in the neuroma following nerve damage in which sprouting occurs in both pain fibers and sympathetic fibers. In experimentally produced neuromas, stimulation of the sympathetic fibers can lead to discharge in the pain fibers. Because pain also can produce sympathetic discharge, the neuroma may produce a positive feedback loop in which sympathetic discharge then leads to further pain impulses (Zimmerman, 1981). Some authors have suggested that this may be part of the mechanism involved in producing tension headaches. This also may be the mechanism for the action of those treatments that use local anesthetic blocks of either the nerve or sympathetic ganglion to interrupt the cycle (Zimmerman, 1981).

At the level of the first synapse there is some evidence to suggest that substance P may be the first transmitter or perhaps acts as a modulator (Terenius, 1981). Glutamate also may act as a transmitter (Terenius, 1981). At the early spinal cord synapse then, there is already evidence for central modulation of the pain impulses.

There have been a number of additional lines of evidence

for a central modulating mechanism of pain impulses. Hypnosis, relaxation, acupuncture, and forms of counterirritation all may produce analgesia through central modulation (Watkins & Mayer, 1982). Electrical stimulation of various brain structures also has been noted to produce analgesia. For example, stimulation of the midbrain at the area of the periaqueductal gray matter can inhibit the firing of the dorsal horn cell neurons (Liebeskind & Paul, 1977). This stimulus-produced analgesia can lead to tolerance similar to the tolerance seen with morphine (Mayer & Hayes, 1975). Stimulus-produced analgesia given together with morphine, with both in suboptimal doses, can lead to analgesia (Samanin & Valzelli, 1971). Stimulus-produced analgesia also produces cross-tolerance with morphine (Mayer & Hayes, 1975). Finally, it has been shown that naloxone can inhibit stimulus-produced analgesia (Akil, Mayer, & Liebeskind, 1976). All of these findings suggest that there are endogenous substances for pain regulation.

Further evidence for the existence of these endogenous substances was provided by the fact that opiate-binding sites can be found in areas that are thought to be related to pain transmission (Watkins & Mayer, 1982). These binding sites are found at several levels, including dorsal horn cells and the periaqueductal gray matter of the midbrain. These binding sites also are found in areas regulating mood and behavior, such as the locus ceruleus and the striatum (Terenius, 1981). Most recently, the endorphins have been identified. They are endogenous substances thought to be naturally occurring opiates. These are found most frequently in the areas where the opiate receptors also are concentrated (Hughes, 1975).

In fact, there are probably a number of inhibitory systems acting at the spinal cord level that are only partially understood. There are also a number of more central systems that are even less well understood.

In addition to the role of the endorphins, two other neuroregulatory systems are also of particular interest because of currently available pharmacological interventions involving these systems. The first of the neurotransmitters is serotonin. Experimentally, decreasing the production of serotonin through the use of agents such as p-chlorophenylalanine can lead to a decrease in the inhibition of pain impulses by stimulus-produced analgesia at the midbrain (Carstens, Fraunhoffer, & Zimmerman, 1981). Since applying morphine at the midbrain produces this inhibition of pain impulses, it is thought that the endorphins produce stimulation of the descending cells from the midbrain that lead to the release of serotonin at the dorsal horn cell (Zimmerman, 1981). Thus, serotonin acts to increase pain impulses in the periphery through its effect on the receptor cells but also acts to inhibit the transmission of pain impulses through its effect on the dorsal horn cells. Tricyclic antidepressants and other serotonergic drugs have clinically been noted to be useful in the treatment of pain syndromes (Murphy & Davis, 1981). This action may in part be due to the effect on this inhibitory system. It also has been suggested that the relationship between chronic pain and depression observed clinically also may have a biochemical link if both chronic pain and depression evoke serotonergic mechanisms (Murphy & Davis, 1981; Zimmerman, 1981).

The second clinically relevant neuroregulatory system is a possible dopamine system. Agents such as the phenothiazines, which block dopamine transmission, have been used in the treatment of chronic pain (Cavenar & Maltbic, 1976). They have been noted to potentiate the effect of narcotic agents (Murphy & Davis, 1981). Conversely, giving l-dopa in some subjects can lead to an increase in sensitivity to pain (Hodge & King, 1976). Haloperidol has been noted to have an effect on the endogenous opiate receptors (Clay & Broughman, 1975). The interaction between the endogenous opiate system and the dopaminergic system is complicated and requires further study. However, manipulation of this system through dopamine blocking agents has already been noted to be clinically useful in many patients with pain.

There is evidence for at least four types of systems involved in the regulation of pain transmission in the central nervous system. There is an apparent neural system involving the endorphins as transmitters. There is also a system in which the endorphins act as hormones rather than as transmitters released into the synapses. There is a neural system that does not involve the endogenous opiates. Finally, there is a hormonal system not involving the endogenous opiate system (Watkins & Mayer, 1982). Thus, it may be possible to find ways of treating patients through a number of these systems sequentially or synergistically to provide more effective pain relief with less risk of addiction (Terenius, 1981; Watkins & Mayer, 1982).

Animal studies have suggested that some of these systems can be influenced by conditioning. In mice a shock to the foot can produce analgesia in the tail. Animals who are exposed to this foot shock in a specific cage will experience the analgesia with the foot shock and will later experience analgesia with exposure to the cage alone without the foot shock (Hayes, Bennett, Newton, & Mayer, 1978). This analgesia can be blocked through the use of narcotic antagonists (Watkins & Mayer, 1982). Thus, it appears that animals can be trained to turn on their endogenous opiate systems.

In addition to studies of the biological mechanisms involved in the transmission of pain impulses, important work has been done in examining physiological responses to pain. Acute pain is generally accomplished by sympathetic adrenergic response with some vagal inhibition. Thus, patients experiencing acute pain are likely to have increases in their heart rate, stroke volume, blood pressure, and respiration (Sternbach, 1968). Patients who experience chronic pain are less likely to have these physiological responses but are more likely to experience physiological changes similar to those seen in depression. Thus, they are described as sleeping less, being more irritable, having less appetite. They are often constipated and frequently withdrawn (Sternbach, 1974). The acute physiological responses have some biological function. They warn of the presence of injury and they enforce some stillness on the individual that allows time for healing. They also assist the individual in coping (Sternbach, 1981). However, after severe injury or surgery, and particularly after severe burns, these physiological changes have little useful function and in fact can lead to many complications from the excess of adrenergic activity and vagal inhibition (Bonica, 1981). In burn patients and surgery patients, recovery is often hindered by the resultant ileus, oliguria, and increased heart work load (Bonica, 1981). The anxiety and adrenergic activity after an acute myocardial infarction has been shown to lead to an increase in the size of the infarct (Zanchetti & Malliani, 1974). It is therefore apparent that proper pain relief, as well as relief of affective components of pain, can be of importance in seriously ill medical patients.

Unfortunately, studies examining the knowledge of physicians regarding the principles of pain relief indicate that many physicians have deficits in their understanding of the principles involved. In one study three-quarters of the patients who were receiving narcotics for severe pain still reported they had moderate to severe pain (Marks & Sachar, 1973). Medical house staff were noted to underestimate the effective dose of pain medication and to overestimate the duration of action. They were also noted to have exaggerated concerns regarding addiction potential and the danger of respiratory complications with pain relief agents (Marks & Sachar, 1973). In fact, pain can be a powerful respiratory stimulant, and this stimulation generally offsets any depression of respiration that occurs with drugs. In addition, drugs for pain can reduce the voluntary muscle immobility seen in pain and thus can lead to better ventilation and a better cough (Bonica, 1981). The risk of narcotic addiction in patients with acute pain is also very small. In one study 1 out of 4,000 patients who received narcotics actually became addicted (Porter & Jick, 1980). Medical patients without serious premorbid psychological difficulties who do become addicted to narcotic agents also generally are easily withdrawn from these agents without further difficulties (Bonica, 1981).

PSYCHOLOGICAL VARIABLES

The psychological investigation of pain has partly involved attempts to quantify pain and to examine psychological variables in relationship to the degree of experimental pain. It is important to remember, however, that experimental pain does not carry the same affective meaning as clinical pain. Thus, it has been difficult to relate experimental studies of pain in the laboratory to the psychological issues seen in patients, particularly patients with chronic pain. There are two commonly measured thresholds for pain. The first of these is the pain threshold in which subjects are asked to report when they first perceive the pain. This initial threshold measure varies little with personality and cultural variables but correlates well with the level of impulses in the sensory neurons. The upper pain threshold is reached when the subject reports that the pain is now unbearable. This upper threshold varies more with age, sex, personality, and other cultural determinants. The difference between the upper and lower thresholds is called the pain tolerance. Pain tolerance is known to vary, particularly with anxiety and with the individual's state of health (Bond, 1981; Ramsey, 1979).

Pain has been studied primarily in relationship to two psychological states—anxiety and depression. In both states the interrelationships are complex, and causality goes in both directions.

Anxiety is associated both physiologically and psychologically with acute pain. Pain can lead to anxiety with all its physiological manifestations, including increased heart rate and blood pressure and dilated pupils (Sternbach, 1981). In Minnesota Multiphasic Personality Inventory (MMPI) studies patients in acute pain demonstrate this anxiety (Sternbach, 1974). Anxiety, on the other hand, also can lead to a decrease in tolerance to pain. Both illness and other environmentally induced anxiety can lead to decreased pain tolerance (Mersky & Spear, 1967). Personality variables known to be related to difficulty in tolerating anxiety such as neuroticism and poor ego strength also have been related to a lessened pain tolerance (Bond, 1973). The effectiveness of anxiety-reducing measures in pain have been fairly well demonstrated. A large component of the effectiveness of prepared childbirth seems to involve anxiety reduction through mechanism involving cognitive preparation (Beck & Siegel, 1980). Anxiolytic agents, relaxation techniques, and various cognitive strategies all can be partially effective in addressing the interaction between anxiety and pain.

Depression correlates with chronic pain more than does anxiety. A number of components of chronically painful conditions would be expected to contribute to the development of a depression. Patients with chronic illness, particularly chronically painful illnesses, experience many losses. These losses include income, independence, effective job functions, mobility, the ability to engage in recreational activities, and a general sense of well-being (Ramsey, 1979). Patients with chronic illnesses tend to experience a sense of helplessness. They see themselves as having little control over their bodies and are often in need of outside assistance for all areas of functioning. They also experience a sense of hopelessness. Chronic pain patients are often described as having no sense of their own ability to change their conditions and also see the doctors as unable to change their conditions. Suicide tends to be more frequent in certain kinds of chronically painful conditions, particularly in older men with intractable pain from cancer (Bond, 1981). It is also more frequent in patients with cluster headaches and in herpetic neuralgias (Bond, 1981).

Depression itself alters a person's response to pain. Some patients with what has been called masked depression present principally with complaints of pain but are thought instead to have primarily a depressive illness (Lesse, 1956). Psychological studies of chronic pain patients without clear lesions suggest that many are depressed (Mersky & Sternbach, 1978). This depends in part on how the depression is measured or defined. One study (Cassidy, Flanagan, Spellman, & Cohen, 1957) looked at the frequency of complaints of pain in patients with depressive illnesses. Pain was not significantly more common in depression than in other psychiatric disorders but was more common than in normal individuals. Blumer & Heilbron (1981) suggested that chronic pain may occur more frequently in families in which there is a history of alcoholism and of unipolar depression. This suggests that some forms of pain syndromes may be a part of the depressive spectrum.

A recent study (Atkinson, Kremer, & Ignelzi, 1982) looked at the language used to describe pain and showed that depressed patients described pain in a more diffuse manner. Thus, in depressed patients descriptions of pain and other symptoms are likely to be less useful diagnostically.

In addition to the relationship between anxiety and depression, there are a number of psychological syndromes and traits that alter pain reports through various mechanisms. George Engel (1959) described a group of patients who he feels are pain-prone. He said that these patients are more likely than others to use pain as a psychic regulator, whether or not the pain includes a peripheral source of stimulation. These pain-prone patients were marked by several features. First, guilt is important in the choice of pain as the symptom, and these individuals were depressed, gloomy, antagonistic, and self-depreciating. Developmentally, these patients' histories were marked by early family relationships in which aggression, suffering, and pain were important. Their pain tended to occur in a number of circumstances. They developed pain when external circumstances failed to satisfy their need to suffer and often followed the achievement of success or good fortune. Pain also occurred as a response to loss or when guilt was evoked by aggressive or forbidden sexual feelings. The location of pain was determined in part by the patient's personal experience with pain or by the pain experienced by, or wished on, another person. These patients had a number of psychiatric diagnoses, including conversion disorders, depression, hypochondriasis, and schizophrenia; some did not fall into any diagnostic category.

The intrapsychic importance of issues of compensation and dependency have been discussed by several authors. The clinical syndrome involving these issues had been called the compensation neurosis. In this syndrome patients are described as dependent, insecure, and needy. However, they tend to conceal these traits by a form of pseudoindependence. They are often described as workaholics, and they have a history of having begun work early, often because of family pressures. With development of pain and injury their long-denied dependency and passivity is aroused. The pain provides a mechanism for continuing this dependency. It also provides a punishment for the dependency and the associated guilt. These patients often are involved in litigation, and the litigation comes to represent payment for the years of toil and suffering that the patient has experienced. Manifest depression tends to be rare during the period of litigation but becomes more apparent after the litigation has been settled (Hackett, 1978).

Issues of self-esteem also are seen as important in influencing pain proneness. This may be in part related to the self-punishing behavior described in pain patients (Blumer & Heilbron,

1981). Using measures of self-esteem, patients with pain beyond that expected in their illness or patients with pain not responding to conventional treatment were found to be low in self-esteem. In the same study, treatment that addressed the difficulty in self-esteem led to a decrease in pain complaints accompanied by an increase in the measure of self-esteem (Elton, Stanley, & Burrows, 1978).

As suggested in the study of psychiatric patients by Cassidy et al. (1957), pain complaints are seen more frequently in a variety of psychiatric disorders. Depression, anxiety disorders, histrionic personalities, hypochondriacal disorders, and schizophrenia are all associated with a greater likelihood of pain complaints (Engel, 1959). However, psychiatric patients have been shown to be more likely to have simultaneously occurring medical illnesses (Amdur & Prizant, 1975), and part of the pain complaints may represent these medical problems.

Numerous studies have examined the psychological characteristics of chronic pain patients. Using the MMPI, Sternbach (1974) showed that in comparison to patients with acute pain, patients with chronic pain have significantly greater elevations on the hypochondriasis and hysteria scales, as well as a greater but slightly less marked elevation on the depression scale. In a later study, Sternbach & Timmermans (1975) demonstrated that when subjects were treated surgically for relief of pain, they had a greater reduction in these MMPI measures than did subjects not treated surgically. However, another study (Naliboff, Cohen, & Yellen, 1982) showed that patients with chronic nonpainful conditions, such as diabetes mellitus and hypertension, had similar elevations. Thus, these elevations may be the effect of chronic illness, and the psychological picture may represent the effect of the chronic limitations of illness. Treatment approaches addressing these limitations but not necessarily addressing the pain directly might benefit both the pain and the emotional distress.

In a study that generated much controversy regarding its interpretation, Timmermans and Sternbach (1974) used factor analytic techniques to study chronic pain patients. The most pertinent personality variable was what they identified as interpersonal alienation and manipulativeness. This personality dimension includes feelings of being out of control of one's life, suspicion and anger toward others, blaming others for one's difficulty, and attempts to manipulate and control others. In response to criticism of the study, the authors argue that this factor has clear implications for the rehabilitation of patients with chronic pain (Timmermans & Sternbach, 1975).

Social Psychology

In addition to the intrapersonal factors involved in the psychology of pain, it is important to consider the interpersonal meaning of pain. Pain has been related to various models drawn from social psychology.

Szasz (1961) suggested there is value in looking at pain not only as a symptom but as a communication, particularly as a communication between the patient and the doctor. He saw some pain as important to the patient in defining himself in the sick role. Complaints of pain are particularly useful as a form of rhetoric, a communication not aimed at explaining something but at convincing someone. Szasz used the term "homodolorosus" (painful man) to describe the person who establishes for himself a role as a professional in pain.

Pilowsky & Spense (1976) expanded on the concept of sick role status to study what they called "abnormal illness behavior." They suggested that since concepts such as conversion and hypochondriasis are hard to define, it may be more useful to think in terms of illness behavior. In a later study, using a measure of abnormal illness behavior, they noted that this measure was more accurate in differentiating chronic pain nonresponders from responders than were measures of depression (Pilowsky, Chapman, & Bonica, 1977). Illness behavior has important interpersonal significance in this model. It can be shown to function in controlling interpersonal relationships, it serves to communicate emotional stress, it can be used to manipulate others, and it can be used to express hostility or to relieve guilt (Pilowsky & Spence, 1976).

This concept has particular relevance in patients with

chronic pain that is not responsive to traditional treatments. Pilowsky and Spence's (1976) study of these patients showed them to have several distinguishing features. In comparison with other chronically ill patients with pain, patients unresponsive to traditional treatments were more convinced of the presence of disease, were more somatically preoccupied, and were less able to accept reassurance from their doctor.

SOCIAL VARIABLES

Several studies have attempted to look at differences between cultural groups in their reaction to pain and pain tolerance. There is little difference in cultural groups in terms of pain thresholds and pain tolerance. However, there do seem to be differences in pain expressiveness (Zborowski, 1969). There are also differences in the affective component of pain. This affective influence includes differences in the autonomic changes that acompany the anxiety of pain (Weisenberg, 1975).

Another social variable that influences pain behavior has been called tertiary gain. Tertiary gain refers to the tendency of families and other social groups to subtly encourage the continuation of pain complaints (Bokan, Ries, & Katon, 1981). Many physicians have encountered marriage partners in which pain in one partner occurs when the alcoholic partner stops drinking. In such situations pain is best considered in terms of its role in the system as a whole.

Pain also can have effects on the social system that have medical relevance. Block's (1981) studies of the spouses of pain patients suggests that pain leads to an altered physiological responsiveness in the spouse. The spouse is seen as being not only more vulnerable to psychological distress but also to physical illness.

Useful work is also being done in looking at the role of patient-staff interactions in hospitals. Pilowsky and Bond (1969) found that on cancer wards those patients who assess themselves as high on pain were more likely to have powerful analgesics withheld by the nursing staff.

THE DISTINCTION BETWEEN PSYCHOGENIC AND PHYSIOLOGIC PAIN

It is clear that in many cases it is important to consider the role of multiple determinants in producing pain complaints. This has led some people to argue against the use of distinctions between psychogenic and "real" pain. This argument has been advanced for a number of reasons.

It has been argued that mind-body dualism ties us to a distinction that is difficult to make and not particularly useful. However, the distinction has persisted, and this may imply that it has some utility for clinicians. Clinicians still wish to identify the nature of the lesion. They feel a need to make targeted rather than shotgun interventions. Psychological intervention also needs to be targeted. The fact is, we cannot always tell what is biological and what is psychological, but there may still be some utility in trying to do so. There is a whole spectrum of ways that pain can arise, both from largely biological and largely psychological mechanisms, and to focus only on the common endpoint, the complaint of pain, weakens our therapeutic armamentarium.

The second argument against the distinction between psychogenic and real pain involves the role of this distinction in producing prejudice. It is argued that considering all pain to be real allows the doctor to treat patients without having to label them as "crocks" or chronic complainers. However, in fact, what this abandoning of the distinction may do would be to allow the doctor to defend against his anger at the patient in ways that may lead to further difficulties. Patients with complaints of intractable pain do often make doctors angry. By denying the existence of differences in pain patients, the doctor may in fact be defending against his anger by altering his usual way of perceiving reality. The psychotherapeutic literature suggests that the doctor who is aware of his anger is less dangerous to the patient than the doctor who denies his anger by distorting reality (Maltsberger & Buie, 1974). Most doctors are, in fact, psychologically healthy enough to say that the patient has no demonstrable lesion but seems to be suffering nonetheless. A doctor can say that the patient may be suffering in a different way and that he would like to help him. Perhaps he may even say to himself and to his colleagues that the patient makes him angry.

The third reason for abandoning the distinction between psychogenic and real pain is that in speaking to patients with pain an approach that acknowledges the reality of pain is more likely to bring the patient in for treatment. However, very often the physician who says he believes a patient's pain is real but also continues to encourage the patient to discuss psychological issues will continue to encounter considerable resistance to further treatment. As was noted previously, many patients with chronic intractable pain seem more interested in convincing the doctor and others of the reality of their pain than in actually getting pain relief. A more useful approach to getting patients into treatment might be to acknowledge the patient's desire to convince the doctor but then to state clearly that the doctor's desire is to help the patient in any way possible. Sternbach (1974) has called this approach interpreting the pain games. Physicians need not be embarrassed about their desire to help the patient with intra- or interpersonal distress, or both.

Thus, it seems that although there may be some reasons for avoiding attempts to divide pain complaints in this way, there are also some risks in doing so. A better approach is probably to acknowledge the complicated nature of pain and our failure at present to understand it fully.

SUMMARY OF TREATMENT CONSIDERATIONS

Each of the various important areas of consideration in understanding pain suggests a number of treatment approaches. Although many of these approaches have been described previously, it is useful to summarize some of the more important treatment considerations.

The multiple biological systems for processing pain information suggest the usefulness of using multiple approaches in the pharmacology of pain relief. Thus, interventions involving serotonin or dopamine should be considered along with interventions involving the prostaglandins and opiates. It is important also to remember that the physiological effects of pain are not always useful. Therefore, active intervention in relieving both the pain and emotional distress is called for. Physicians have a history of undertreating acute pain and overtreating chronic pain.

Psychological interventions involve actively looking for and attending to the accompanying anxiety or depression. Knowledge of the psychological syndromes that can produce complaints of pain can lead to more rapid treatment of these specific syndromes. Issues of masochism and guilt, impaired ability to maintain self-esteem, dependency, and litigation also should be evaluated.

The role of the symptom as a communication also should be considered. Treament can thus be focused on allowing the patient to communicate in other ways. Particular attention should be paid to those patients who seem excessively convinced of their disease, who seem more interested in convincing their doctor, and who are not able to accept reassurance. The need for the family to maintain the symptom and the effects of the pain on the social system also should be evaluated.

Attention to all of these factors can be very time-consuming. Pain centers may be partially successful because they expect to spend time and effort in obtaining a full evaluation of all components of the pain complaints. However, it is far easier for the average physician practicing alone simply to write a prescription. Working with pain patients also can be very frustrating. Often, what is done is not as important as what is not done. Thus, identifying those patients who should not receive active surgical or medical interventions is particularly important.

A strategy for preventing the development of chronic pain in patients with acute pain also should be considered. DeFelice and Sunshine (1981) have suggested several elements of such a strategy. Patients who are most vulnerable need to be recognized. The doctor should make clear statements regarding the expected course and the use of drugs, so that patients know that pain relief will be provided on a temporary basis. Patients should be given appointments for return visits at a specified time, so that they don't need to justify a visit to the doctor. Finally, any increase in medication consumption or decrease in activity when the patient should be feeling better signals a need to reevaluate the treatment program.

REFERENCES

Akil, H., Mayer, D.J., & Liebeskind, J.C. (1976). Antagonism of stimulation-produced analgesia by naloxone, a narcotic antagonist. *Science, 191,* 961–962.

Amdur, M.A., & Prizant, G. (1975). Health care issues in a psychiatric aftercare program. *Psychosomatics, 16,* 155–160.

Atkinson, J. H., Kremer, E. F., & Ignelzi, R. J. (1982). Diffusion of pain language with affective disturbance confounds differential diagnosis. *Pain, 12,* 375–384.

Beck, N.C., & Siegel, L. J. (1980). Preparation for childbirth and contemporary research on pain, anxiety, and stress reduction: A review and critique. *Psychosomatic Medicine, 42,* 429–447.

Beecher, H. K. (1959). *Measure of subjective responses.* New York: Oxford University Press.

Block, A. R. (1981). An investigation of the response of the spouse to chronic pain behavior. *Psychosomatic Medicine, 43,* 415–422.

Blumer, D., & Heilbronn, M. (1981). The pain-prone disorder: A clinical and psychological profile. *Psychosomatics, 22,* 395–402.

Bokan, J. A., Ries, R. K., & Katon, W. J. (1981). Tertiary gain and chronic pain. *Pain, 10,* 331–335.

Bond, M. R. (1973). Personality studies in patients with pain secondary to organic disease. *Journal of Psychosomatic Research, 17,* 257–263.

Bond, M. R. (1981). Patients' experience of pain. *Pharmacology and Therapeutics, 12,* 563–573.

Bonica, J. J. (1981). [Editorial]. *Triangle, 20,* 1–6.

Carstens, E., Fraunhoffer, M., & Zimmerman, M. (1981). Serotonergic mediation of descending inhibition from midbrain periaqueductal grey, but not reticular formation of spinal nociceptive transmission in the cat. *Pain, 10,* 149–167.

Cassidy, W. L., Flanagan, N. B., Spellman, B. A., & Cohen, M. E. (1957). Clinical observations in manic-depressive disease: A quantitative study of one hundred manic-depressive patients and 50 medically sick controls. *Journal of American Medical Association, 164,* 1535–1546.

Cavenar, J. D., & Maltbic, A. A. (1976). Another indication for haloperidol. *Psychosomatics, 17,* 128–130.

Clay, G. S., & Broughman, L. R. (1975). Haloperidol binding to an opiate receptor site. *Biochemical Pharmacology, 24,* 1363–1367.

DeFelice, E. A., & Sunshine, A. (1981). Basic principles in the management of pain. *Triangle, 20,* 43–48.

Elton, D., Stanley, G. V., & Burrows, G.D. (1978). Self-esteem and chronic pain. *Journal of Psychosomatic Research, 22,* 25–30.

Engel, G. L. (1959). Psychogenic pain and the pain-prone patient. *American Journal of Medicine, 26,* 899–918.

Engel, G. L. (1977). The need for a new medical model: A challenge for biomedicine. *Science, 196,* 129–136.

Hackett, T. P. (1978). The pain patient: Evaluation and treatment. In T. P. Hackett & N. H. Cassem, (Eds.), *Massachusetts General Hospital handbook of general hospital psychiatry.* (pp. 41–63) St. Louis: C. V. Mosby.

Hayes, R. L., Bennett, G. L., Newton, P. G., & Mayer, D. J. (1978). Behavioral and physiological studies of non-narcotic analgesia in the rate elicited by certain environmental stimuli. *Brain Research, 155,* 69–90.

Hodge, C. J., & King, R. B. (1976). Medical modification of sensation. *Journal of Neurosurgery, 44,* 21–28.

Hughes, J. (1975). Isolation of an endogenous compound from the brain with pharmacological properties similar to morphine. *Brain Research, 88,* 295–308.

IASP Subcommittee on Taxonomy. Pain terms: A list with definitions and notes on usage. *Pain, 6,* 249–252.

Lesse, S. (1956). Atypical facial pain syndromes of psychogenic origin: Complications of their misdiagnosis. *Journal of Nervous Mental Disorders, 124,* 346.

Liebeskind, J. C., & Paul, L. A. (1977). Psychological and physiological mechanisms of pain. *Annual Review of Psychology, 28,* 41–60.

Maltsberger, J. T., & Buie, D. H. (1974). Countertransference hate in the treatment of suicidal patients. *Archives of General Psychiatry, 30,* 625–633.

Marks, R.M., & Sachar, E. J. (1973). Undertreatment of medical patients with narcotic analgesics. *Annals of Internal Medicine, 78,* 173–181.

Mayer, D. J., & Hayes, R. L. (1975). Stimulation-produced analgesia: Development of tolerance and cross-tolerance to morphine. *Science, 188,* 941–943.

Merskey, H. (1978) Pain and personality. In R. A. Sternbach, (Ed)., *The psychology of pain.* (pp. 111–127) New York: Raven Press.

Merskey, H., & Spear, F. G. (1967). *Pain: Psychological and psychiatric aspects.* London: Bailiere, Tindall and Cassell.

Murphey, M. F., & Davis, K. L. (1981). Biological perspectives in chronic pain, depression, and organic mental disorders. *Psychiatric Clinics of North America, 4,* 223-238.

Naliboff, B. D., Cohen, M. J., & Yellen, A. N. (1982). Does the MMPI differentiate chronic illness from chronic pain? *Pain, 13,* 333–341.

Pilowski, I., & Bond, M. R. (1969). Pain and its management in malignant disease. *Psychosomatic Medicine, 31,* 400–404.

Pilowski, I., Chapman, C. R., & Bonica, J. J. (1977). Pain, depression, and illness behavior in a pain clinic population. *Pain, 4,* 183–192.

Pilowski, I., & Spence, N. D. (1976). Pain and illness behavior: A comparative study. *Journal of Psychosomatic Research, 20,* 131–134.

Porter, J., & Jick, H. (1980). Addiction rare in patients treated with narcotics. *New England Journal of Medicine, 302,* 123.

Ramsey, R. A. (1979). The understanding and teaching of reaction to pain. *Bibliotheca Psychiatrica, 159,* 114–140.

Samanin, R., & Valzelli, L. (1971). Increase of morphine-induced analgesia by stimulation of the nucleus raphe dorsalis. *European Journal of Pharmacology, 16,* 298–302.

Sternbach, R. A. (1968). *Pain: A psychophysiological analysis.* New York: Academic Press.

Sternbach, R. A. (1974). *Pain patients: Traits and treatment.* New York: Academic Press.

Sternbach, R. A. (1981). Chronic pain as a disease entity. *Triangle, 20,* 27–32.

Sternbach, R. A., & Timmermans, G. (1975). Personality changes associated with reduction of pain. *Pain, 1,* 177–181.

Szasz, T. S. (1957). *Pain and pleasure: A study of bodily feelings.* New York: Basic Books.

Szasz, T. S. (1961). *The myth of mental illness: Foundations of a theory of personal conduct.* New York: Harper.

Terenius, L. (1981). Biochemical mediators in pain. *Triangle, 20,* 19–26.

Timmermans, G., & Sternbach, R. A. (1974). Factors of human chronic pain: An analysis of personality and pain reaction variables. *Science, 184,* 806–808.

Timmermans, G., & Sternbach, R. A. (1975). Analysis of human chronic pain. *Science, 187,* 861–862.

Watkins, L. R., & Mayer, D. J. (1982). Organization of opiate and non-opiate pain control systems. *Science, 216,* 1185–1192.

Weisenberg, M. (1975). *Pain: Clinical and experimental perspectives.* St. Louis: C. V. Mosby.

Zanchetti, A., & Malliani, A. (1974). Neural and psychological factors in coronary disease. *Acta Cardiologica, 20* (Suppl.), 69–93.

Zborowski, M. (1969). *People in pain.* San Francisco: Jossey-Bass.

Zimmerman, M. (1981). Physiological mechanisms of pain and pain therapy. *Triangle, 20,* 7–18.

Chapter 5

SLEEP IN VARIOUS MEDICAL AND SURGICAL CONDITIONS

Constance A. Moore, Ismet Karacan, and Robert L. Williams

Sleep research has burgeoned over the last three decades, particularly since the discovery of rapid eye movement (REM) sleep. At first, sleep research focused on definitions of what constituted normal sleep and speculation about the purpose of sleep. Later, studies of the primary sleep disorders and physiological functioning in sleep were central. More recently, neurotransmitters' role in sleep and sleep in various medical and surgical conditions have been studied.

It has long been believed that adequate sleep is necessary for good health and recovery from illness. However, there has been far too little documentation of these beliefs. This chapter reviews the literature on sleep in a variety of medical and surgical conditions, focusing primarily on the effects of the conditions on sleep and the effects of sleep on these disorders. The latter is an area that for the most part continues to be an enigma.

SLEEP AND CARDIOVASCULAR FUNCTION

There have been a number of studies of cardiovascular function in the sleep of animals and man (Coccagna, Mantovani, Brignani, Manzini, Lugaresi, 1971; Gauzzi, Bacelli & Zanchetti, 1968; Guazzi & Zanchetti, 1965; Khatri & Freis, 1967; Mancia, Bacelli, Adams, & Zanchetti, 1971; Miller & Helander, 1979). The major findings follow.

Heart rate (HR) and blood pressure (BP) fall during non-REM (NREM) sleep and reach their lowest and least variable values in slow-wave sleep (SWS). During REM sleep, mean arterial BP and HR do not fall below NREM values; instead there is an increased variability of these measures that coincides with REM phasic events. In short, there is a tonic decrease in BP and HR with superimposed phasic increases in BP and brief tachycardia in REM sleep. There may be a following rebound bradycardia. The parasympathetic nervous system is mainly responsible for the bradycardia in sleep, with a lesser role ascribed to decreased sympathetic tone. Hypertensive patients have falls in BP in sleep that may be greater in amplitude but similar in percentage of decrease to those seen in normotensive subjects.

Cardiac output falls in NREM sleep and is lowest in REM sleep in animals; there is an overall increased peripheral resistance, with regional differences (dilation of mesenteric and renal vessels and constriction of the external iliac artery). Cardiac output and peripheral resistance decrease in human sleep as well, and there are episodes of vasoconstriction that occur during REM phasic events.

Because of the transient increases in BP, HR, and vasoconstriction that occur during REM sleep, many researchers have speculated that these may be related to the reported increase of myocardial infarction, angina, and dysrhythmias during sleep.

Dysrhythmias

There are many case reports of cardiac patients suffering either increased arrhythmias or arrhythmias occurring exclusively in sleep. These include premature ventricular contractions (PVCs), premature atrial beats, tachy- and bradycardias, bigeminy, and others.

Rosenblatt, Hartmann, and Azillig (1973) studied 10 patients with PVCs for a total of 30 nights and found PVCs most often in REM sleep, then in stages 4, 2, and 3, respectively. Eight patients had had previous myocardial infarctions, and none were receiving antiarrhythmic drugs. In a study of 28 "asymptomatic" patients with PVCs, Regestein, DeSilva, and Lown (1981) found the frequency of PVCs increased during REM sleep compared with other sleep stages, an increase that was independent of HR. However, a study of 48 patients with coronary artery disease, 24 medically treated and 24 who had had bypass surgery, revealed no significant differences in the number of PVCs between REM and NREM sleep (Karacan, Guinn, et al., 1977).

Monti et al. (1975), studying 10 patients with arrhythmias and coronary artery disease, and Smith, Johnson, Rothfeld, Zir, and Tharp (1972), monitoring 18 patients with dysrhythmias, admitted to the coronary care unit (7 on antiarrythmic drugs), also found no differences in the frequency of PVCs in REM versus NREM sleep. Monti et al. (1975) found a temporal relationship between dysrhythmias and sleep stage in some patients, but when patients were considered as a group, no significant correlation could be observed. The patients of Smith et al. (1972) (44 percent with acute myocardial infarction, 39 percent with chronic cardiac disease, and 17 percent with other or unknown diagnoses) had a nonsignificant tendency for increased PVCs during sleep-wake transitions compared to the number occurring during sleep stage transitions.

We know of only a single 24-h study of heart rhythm in patients with heart disease (Lown, Tykocinski, Garfein, & Brooks, 1973). Fifty-four ambulatory patients were evaluated, 31 with coronary artery disease, 11 with miscellaneous heart ailments, and 12 without known organic heart disease but with dizziness, palpitations, and syncope. Electroencephalographic (EEG) and electro-oculographic (EOG) monitoring were not done. Forty-five patients showed some PVCs during the 24-h monitoring sessions: 78 percent of these had a decrease in ectopic activity during sleep, and about half of those with decreased number of PVCs had a decrease of 50 percent or more. Seven of the 12 subjects with symptoms but without known heart disease had PVCs. Four of the seven had had a decrease of PVCs during sleep. Unfortunately, the lack of EEG/EOG monitoring to distinguish sleep from nocturnal waking, sleep-waking transitions, and sleep stages makes it impossible to relate arrhythmias to these phases of sleep.

Patients with congenital heart block (CHB) also have been studied. Twenty CHB patients had nocturnal Holter monitoring (Levy, Camm, & Keane, 1977). The most notable finding was that 35 percent of the patients showed marked ventricular slowing during sleep (RR intervals of 3,000 to 6,000 ms). Most of the sudden RR-interval prolongations were 2:1 or 3:1 exit block of the junctional focus.

Four mitral valve prolapse outpatients who had Holter monitor–documented nocturnal arrhythmias were studied polysomnographically by Orr, Langevin, and Stahl (1977). One patient was taking medication: diazepam, phenytoin, and propranolol. There was no significant difference in the rate of occurrence of arrhythmias across sleep stages.

Thus, despite the many case reports of increased arrhythmias during sleep, the one available 24-h ECG study of a large sample of patients revealed a mean decrease in arrhythmias during sleep (Lown et al., 1973). However, individual patients nevertheless may have increased ectopic activity that may be related to sleep-stage or sleep-waking transition. There have not been consistent findings concerning sleep-stage relatedness or arrhythmias. Two studies have found increased PVCs during REM as compared to NREM sleep (Regestein et al., 1981; Rosenblatt et al., 1973); others have not (Karacan, Guinn, et al., 1977; Monti et al., 1975; Orr et al., 1977; Smith et al., 1972). Possible reasons for the differing results are the differences in subject selection and clinical diagnoses of patients both within a given study and across studies.

Nocturnal Angina

As with arrhythmias, researchers have speculated about the possible relationship between REM sleep, with its autonomic activity bursts, and nocturnal angina. In 1923 MacWilliams proposed that dreams cause heightened emotional and physiological states that could give rise to angina. He also observed that deaths from cardiovascular disorders occurred often between 5 and 6 a.m., when REM sleep is more prominent. To test this hypothesis Nowlin et al. (1965) polysomnographically studied four patients with angina. They found a correlation between REM sleep and ST-segment depression, which is associated with ischemia, on the ECG. Of 39 episodes of nocturnal angina 82 percent were associated with REM sleep.

Stern and Tzivoni (1973) performed 24-h Holter monitoring without EEG/EOG on 140 patients with ischemic heart disease and 42 normal subjects. Of the 97 patients with fixed abnormal ST changes during the day, 40 percent had decreased, 36 percent had no change, and 24 percent had increased severity of ST-segment conformation. The authors propose decreased myocardial oxygen demands as a reason for improved ECG in the first group. No explanation was offered for deterioration of ST-segment conformation in the latter group.

There has been at least one study of the effects of nocturnal angina on sleep. Karacan, Williams, and Taylor (1969) studied 10 patients with a history of nocturnal angina. The sleep of these patients was disturbed. Sleep-onset latency was increased, and sleep efficiency was decreased. SWS decreased, and nocturnal awakenings (stage 0) and NREM light sleep (stages 1 and 2) were increased. Subjective reports of pain were associated with only 8 percent of awakenings.

In summary, the available data leave unanswered the question of whether nocturnal angina is related to sleep stage. One study (Nowlin et al., 1965) suggests that cardiac ischemia and angina are related to REM sleep but included only four subjects. Ischemic changes on ECG in angina patients can either improve, worsen, or remain the same (Stern & Tzivoni, 1973), and sleep is disturbed in patients with a history of nocturnal angina compared with controls (Karacan, Williams, & Taylor 1969), whether they are experiencing pain or not.

SLEEP AND THE INTENSIVE CARE UNIT

Not suprisingly, patients in intensive care units (ICUs) suffer sleep deprivation. The noise, lights, devices attached to the patient, drugs, and the anxiety, depression, and pain caused by serious illness can all contribute to sleep disturbance. Sleep deprivation is known to disrupt mental and physical functioning (Gunderson, Dunne, & Feyer, 1973; Johnson, 1969; Passouant, Cadilhac, Baldy-Moulinier, & Mion, 1966; Sassin, 1970), and some authors attribute impaired healing and "ICU psychoses" to sleep deprivation (Dlin, Rosen, Dickstein, Lyons, & Fisher, McFadden & Giblin, 1971), although there is no direct evidence for these relationships. Several studies have addressed the quality of sleep in the ICU.

Karacan, Green, et al. (1973) monitored four myocardial infarction patients continuously from day 2 through day 6 following admission to the ICU. Sleep disruption was remarkable. No patient had stage 3 or 4 sleep; two had no REM sleep during the 120-h continuous monitoring per patient! Of course, other sleep parameters were abnormal: sleep efficiency, percentage of REM sleep, and number of REM periods were decreased: percentage of stage 0 sleep was increased; total time asleep (TST) was 10 to 12h. Stages 1 and 2 sleep percentages were variable. There was a partial breakdown of the circadian sleep-wake cycle.

Another study of post-myocardial-infarction patients in an ICU revealed less dramatic results but again very depressed SWS and REM sleep (Broughton & Baron, 1973).

There is one study of five pre- and post-heart-valve-replacement patients (Elwell, Frankel, & Snyder, 1974). Patients were studied for 4 nights after transfer from the recovery room. No patient had SWS either before or after surgery, and there was no REM sleep while patients were in the recovery room. The postoperative results are consistent with those of Karacan, Green, et al. (1973) in myocardial infarction patients and demonstrate severe sleep disturbance in medical and surgical patients in the ICU. Disturbed sleep in heart surgery patients can last up to at least 5 weeks postoperatively (Orr & Stahl, 1977).

SLEEP AND RESPIRATION

This area, in particular the sleep apnea syndromes, has been the most extensively studied of the sleep disorders. Normal respiratory function during sleep also has been relatively well studied. We will begin with a discussion of normal respiratory physiology in sleep, which will serve as a basis for understanding respiratory dysfunction in sleep.

Normal Respiratory Function in Sleep

Sleep is a time of decreased respiratory function in normal subjects. Wakefulness itself is a stimulus to breathing (Fink, 1961). In SWS, respiratory rate and minute ventilation decrease, breathing depth is very regular, arterial carbon dioxide pressure increases, and the sensitivity of the ventilatory response to carbon dioxide is decreased in comparison to waking (Sullivan, 1980). Lung secretions are retained due to increased mucociliary clearance (Bateman, Clarke, Pavia, & Sheahan, 1978), and in dogs coughing does not occur in either NREM or REM sleep. Further reducing respiratory function is the partial collapse of the upper airway as a result of decreased smooth muscle tone in REM and NREM sleep and the hypotonia of intercostal, geniogossal, and other upper airway muscles in REM sleep (Fink, 1961). All of these changes in function are of no clinical consequence in normal subjects but can detrimentally affect patients with already impaired pulmonary function.

Nocturnal Asthma

There are only a limited number of studies of asthma in sleep, and it is unclear whether the incidence of asthmatic attacks is generally increased in sleep, although many individuals complain that it is. Lowest peak respiratory flow rates in asthma patients have been found at night (Turner-Warwick, 1977). There is some controversy as to whether the reduced flow rates are due to time of day (Hetzel & Clark, 1979) or are more sleep-dependent (Clark & Hetzel, 1977). Further complicating the question of whether sleep per se accounts for increased incidence of asthmatic attacks is the fact that inhaled histamine (a bronchoconstrictor) has more effect in the supine than in the upright position (Bonhuye, 1963). Other explanations for circadian variations in asthma are the cyclic occurrence of cholinesterase, which breaks down acetylcholine (Criep, 1969), a nocturnal increase in sensitivity to histamine (de Vries, Goei, Booy-Noord, & Orie, 1962), reduction of sympathetic tone at night (Soutar, Carruthers, & Pickering, 1977), increase in vagal tone (Soutar et al., 1977), and diminished levels of corticosteroids (Nichols & Tyler, 1967).

There have been several studies of whether nocturnal asthma is related to sleep stage. A study of three asthmatic patients monitored for 21 subject nights reported that 54 percent of attacks occurred in REM sleep and almost no attacks occurred in SWS (Ravenscroft & Hartmann, 1968). Kales and colleagues (Kales, Beall, Bajor, Jacobson, & Kales, 1968; Kales, Kales, & Sly, 1973) have studied both asthmatic adults and children. Twelve adults monitored for 35 subject nights revealed no association between asthmatic attacks and sleep stage or time of night, except that attacks were less frequent in the first hour of the night. In 10 children monitored for 25 subject nights there were no attacks during the first third of the night, when SWS predominates, and 10 episodes each in the middle and last thirds of the night. The sleep of both the adults and the children was disturbed, with decreased stage 4 sleep and TST and increased number of awakenings. The authors suggest that fewer attacks occur during SWS because the depth of the sleep prevents awakening or because there is a decrease in "respiratory difficulty" in SWS. Studies of normal respiratory function in sleep, however, indicate that arousal in response to airway occlusion, hypoxia, hypercapnia, and irritation is more rapid in NREM sleep than in REM sleep (Sullivan, 1980). The possibility of a decrease in "respiratory difficulty" in SWS is difficult to assess. Minute ventilation and respiratory rates in normals decrease in SWS compared with light sleep (LS) or REM sleep, muscle tone shows a decrease from waking and increase above REM sleep levels, and rate and depth of respiration are very stable.

Other Chronic Lung Disease and Sleep

Sleep and chronic obstructive lung disease are mutually exacerbating conditions. That is, respiratory difficulty can disturb sleep, and sleep can worsen pulmonary function, leading to hypoxia, hypercapnia, and apnea. Nocturnal hypoxia can lead to cardiac arrhythmias (Flick & Block, 1979) and eventually can contribute to cor pulmonale. Seven emphysema patients with normal resting awake carbon dioxide tensions and arterial oxygen saturations of less than 96 percent all showed decreased oxygen saturation during sleep (Trask & Cree, 1962). In another study with polysomnography (Koo, Sax, & Snider, 1975) 15 patients with chronic obstructive lung disease were compared to controls and found to have decreased arterial oxygen partial pressures (Pa_{O2}). The fall in Pa_{O2} and the rise in Pa_{CO2} occurred with sleep onset and showed little fluctuation during stages 1, 2, and 3. During REM sleep rapid increases in hypoxemia and hypercapnia occurred. Changes in arterial blood gases tended to be greater in similar stages of sleep as the night wore on.

Pulmonary artery pressures during sleep were monitored without EEG by Vogel, Kelminson, and Cotton (1967) in seven patients with reactive pulmonary hypertension due to intracardiac shunts or chronic obstructive lung disease. During sleep there was an increase of 21 mm Hg in mean pressure, associated with blood gas changes. This causes increased load on the right ventricle and perhaps hastens cor pulmonale in such patients.

To summarize, sleep leads to a reduction in pulmonary function in terms of minute ventilation, response to hypoxia and hypercapnia, mucus clearance, and smaller upper airway caliber. Not surprisingly, patients with chronic obstructive lung disease suffer even greater compromise of respiratory function in sleep, and pulmonary hypertension can be exacerbated. The available data do not indicate any clear sleep stage relationship to nocturnal asthma, although it may be more frequent in REM sleep and less frequent in SWS. The latter would be consistent with the findings of greater constriction of the upper airway during REM sleep. And finally, respiratory difficulty during sleep leads to disturbed sleep and complaints of insomnia. Treatment of the insomnia with hypnotics is not recommended because of the possibility of decreased respiratory drive.

SLEEP APNEA SYNDROMES

Apnea is the cessation of air exchange at the nose and mouth for at least 10 s. A diagnosis of sleep apnea syndrome requires at least 30 such episodes during 7 h of sleep. Apneic episodes occurring solely at the transition from wakefulness to sleep and during eye movement bursts in REM sleep are generally not considered pathological because they occur in normal subjects. Sleep apnea is considered a primary sleep disorder when it is unassociated with respiratory dysfunction during waking. We will define and briefly discuss the primary sleep apneas, but in keeping with the focus of this chapter, our main interest is in the secondary sleep respiratory disorders—those associated with other medical conditions.

Sleep apnea syndromes (SAS) can be classified into three types: (1) upper airway or obstructive sleep apnea, (2) central sleep apnea, and (3) mixed sleep apnea. Upper airway sleep apnea is characterized by cessation of air flow at the nose and mouth but continued diaphragmatic and respiratory muscle efforts. In central sleep apnea respiratory efforts cease temporarily, and in mixed sleep apnea there is an initial central apnea followed by resumption of respiratory efforts against a temporarily blocked upper airway. During apneic spells arterial oxygen saturation can fall below 50 percent. Apnea can occur during any stage of sleep but in some patients is found predominantly concentrated in REM or NREM sleep. Patients with severe SAS can suffer hundreds of apneic episodes per night.

SAS is much more common in men than in women (10–30:1) and occurs most frequently in the fifth and sixth decades of life. Patients with upper airway SAS and mixed SAS are frequently obese or have anatomical causes for the upper airway obstruction. These patients snore loudly and fitfully. Other complaints are excessive daytime sleepiness, abnormal motor movements in sleep, automatic behavior diurnally, hypnogogic hallucinations, personality and intellectual deterioration, headaches, and other symptoms. Central SAS patients may have excessive daytime sleepiness but often complain instead of insomnia or many nocturnal awakenings. Snoring and abnormal motor movements in sleep are not particularly noted.

Treatment of patients with upper airway and mixed apnea is most commonly diet and/or tracheostomy. Removal of large tonsils, adenoids, or other obstructions relieves apnea in some patients. At present there is no well-established treatment for patients with central SAS. There are case reports of improvement with chlorimipramine hydrochloride and doxepin hydrochloride (Guilleminault & Dement, 1978), and with diaphragm pacemaker (Glenn, Holcomb, Shaw, Hogan, & Halschuh, 1976).

SLEEP AND GASTROINTESTINAL DISORDERS

Reflux Esophagitis

Esophageal dysfunction is important in the pathogenesis of reflux esophagitis, and this has been the focus of several investigations. Gastroesophageal reflux in the supine position occurs more frequently in patients with esophagitis than in normals (DeMeester & Johnson, 1975; Johnson & DeMeester, 1974). Since swallowing occurs much less frequently during sleep (Lichter & Muir, 1975) and since patients with esophagitis require more swallows to clear refluxed acid (Booth, Kemmerer, & Skinner, 1968), acid contact with mucosa is much longer during sleep. Increased acid contact time is a known causative factor in esophagitis. Further, Johnson, DeMeester, and Haggitt (1978) have suggested a relationship between severe forms of esophagitis and the frequency of supine reflux. Thus, sleep and a supine position clearly exacerbate this condition.

Duodenal Ulcer Disease

Excesses of gastric acid secretion are related to duodenal ulcer disease. However, few good studies have been done investigating gastric acid secretion in sleep in normal and ulcer patients. Stacher (1975) studied acid secretion in four healthy females and concluded that it decreases with increasing depth of sleep and is decreased overall below waking values; another publication states that patients with duodenal ulcers secrete 3 to 20 times the gastric acid during sleep that normals do (Dragstedt, 1959). However, neither statement can be considered conclusive in view of the multiple methodological problems.

Orr, Hall, Stahl, Durkin, and Whitsett (1976) remotely sampled gastric contents every 20 min and found less inhibition of acid secretion during the first 2 h of sleep in ulcer patients compared with normals. There was much inter- and intranight variation. Clearly, further study with improved technology and methodologies is indicated to gain an understanding of possible effects of sleep on duodenal ulcer disease.

What about the intriguing idea that gastrointestinal function affects the sleep-waking cycle? Kukorelli and Juhasz (1978) found that electrical and mechanical stimulation of cat intestine and splanchnic nerve induced cortical synchronization. Further, SWS and increased number of paradoxical sleep episodes (analogous to REM sleep) were induced by intestinal stimulation (Kukorelli & Juhasz, 1977). They discuss evidence that secretin and cholecystokin may be involved in this effect.

SLEEP AND HEPATIC ENCEPHALOPATHY

Encephalopathies can lead to disturbed sleep-waking cycle, with increased daytime sleep and nocturnal sleep disturbance. Systematic 24-h EEG studies of patients with hepatic encephalopathy are not available. However, Bergonzi, Bianco, Mazza, and Mennuni (1978) have monitored nocturnal sleep in 25 patients with severe hepatic failure. Patients show multiple awakenings, increased stage 0 sleep, global diminution of sleep stages, and particularly, reduced stage REM sleep. There was a relatively high incidence of stages 3 and 4 sleep, which was explained by the high incidence of slow activity in the EEG tracings of encephalopathic patients. Lactulose therapy led to an improvement toward more normal sleep patterns. It is not known whether the decreases in total sleep time and the global diminution of the stages of sleep would be found if patients were monitored over a 24-h period.

SLEEP AND GENITOURINARY CONDITIONS

Menstrual Cycles and Sleep

There have been several reports of recurring hypersomnias associated with menstruation or the end of the menstrual cycle. The best-documented case study is of a thirteen-year-old female (Billiard, Guilleminault, & Dement, 1975). TST averaged approximately 14⅓ h day, and waking EEG showed low-amplitude amorphous theta and asymmetry with right-sided low-amplitude background during a hypersomnia episode. An EEG during an episode without hypersomnia showed some improvement.

After probenicid, 5-hydroxyindoleacetic acid (5-HIAA), a metabolite of serotonin, abnormally increased, suggesting an increased turnover of serotonin. Serotonin is believed to be essentially involved in the regulation of NREM sleep.

Treatment with Premarin® (conjugated estrogens, equine), which blocks secretion of progesterone, eliminated the hypersomnia episodes; progesterone can induce sleep in humans. Hartmann (1966) polysomnographically studied five women during a total of 92 nights to find any sleep architecture changes associated with the menstrual cycle. There was a tendency toward increased REM sleep time late in the menstrual cycle. TST was unchanged.

PREGNANCY AND SLEEP

Sleep has been shown to be disturbed throughout pregnancy (Karacan & Williams, 1970). There are significantly increased TST and more napping in early pregnancy than in nonpregnant controls. TST reaches normal levels in the second trimester and then falls to subnormal levels. The number of awakenings increases and stage 4 sleep markedly decreases in the third trimester. Stage 4 sleep rebounds about 4 to 6 weeks postpartum.

RENAL DISEASE AND SLEEP

In humans, urine volume and excretion of sodium, potassium, chloride, and calcium decrease during sleep (Rubin, 1980). There are decreased urine volume and increased osmolality during REM sleep compared with the other sleep stages (Mandell et al., 1966). Plasma renin activity also decreases in REM sleep (Mullen, James, Lightman, Linsell, & Peart, 1980).

According to Passouant et al. (1970), uremic patients obtain less TST and SWS, and their REM-NREM cycles are less organized than in normals. A study (Karacan, Williams, Bose, Hursch, & Warson, 1972) of 10 patients on chronic hemodialysis revealed that there was increased stage 0 sleep and decreased sleep efficiency on the night preceding dialysis compared with the controls. After dialysis there were decreased TST and stage 4 sleep and increased percentage of stage 0 sleep. Posttransplant patients also have disturbed sleep (Karacan, Williams, Bose, et al., 1972). Polysomnographic studies of nine patients, one studied 5 years postoperatively and eight studied from 3 to 6 months postoperatively, revealed increased percentage of stage 0 sleep and decreased TST and percentage of stage 4 sleep. Both dialysis and transplant patients had the following qualitative sleep EEG changes: decreased number, duration, and quality of spindles; deterioration of K-complexes; increased theta activity, decreased delta wave voltage; and intermingled alpha activity with other frequencies. These and the sleep stage findings are nonspecific abnormalities that are evidence of disturbed brain function in sleep. The etiology of these changes is not known but could be related to medications, to neurologic damage occurring in uremia that does not reverse early post transplant, or to other known factors.

MUSCULOSKELETAL DISORDERS AND SLEEP

Concern about sleep disturbances in patients with musculoskeletal disorders has focused on three areas: (1) insomnia due to pain and stiffness, (2) sleep-respiratory impairment due to skeletal deformity, and (3) sleep disturbance leading to the development of pain and/or stiffness.

The first of these propositions, that insomnia is due to pain and stiffness in rheumatic conditions, has intuitive appeal and is supported by anecdotal evidence. However, we know of no systematic study that objectively evaluates the effects of pain and/or stiffness on sleep. Condie (1979) conducted a questionnaire study of 61 patients "with symptomatic degenerative joint disease causing sleeplessness." Sleep was subjectively improved with the use of an antianxiety agent, chlormezanone. Unfortunately, this study provides little information about the etiology, quality, and severity of sleep disturbance and assumes initially that pain and stiffness cause insomnia.

Mezon, West, Israels, and Kayger (1980) polysomnographically studied two women and three men with severe kyphoscoliosis. They found a spectrum of sleep breathing abnormalities "ranging from no abnormalities to prolonged periods of severe central apnea in two patients." In both patients the apneas were almost entirely associated with REM sleep. The two women had no apneic episodes. Eighty percent of patients had significantly lower mean arterial oxygen saturations (Sa_{O2}) during REM sleep than during waking, and in all patients the lowest Sa_{O2} of the night occurred during REM sleep. Because there were no controls provided and polysomnography was done only one night for some patients, the effect of the severe kyphoscoliosis with respiratory impairment on sleep architecture is difficult to assess.

Moldofsky, Scarisbrick, England, and Smythe (1975) have viewed the problem of sleep disturbance and musculoskeletal disorder from another perspective. As they state, "Traditionally, it has been assumed that pain causes sleep disturbance"; they evaluate instead the possibility of a sleep disturbance leading to increased pain and stiffness. Ten patients with "fibrositis syndrome" were studied over 2 to 3 nights of sleep. Fibrositis syndrome is a group of painful disorders in which, unlike many musculoskeletal disorders, "definitive physical pathology has not been found to be associated with localized areas of non-articular pain and stiffness characteristic of the disorder." Generally, the disorder does not respond to most medical and psychiatric therapies. The authors evaluated sleep stages, investigator-rated patient mood pre- and post-sleep, dolorimeter measurements of musculoskeletal pain, and subjective reports of the presence and intensity of symptoms. All patients had a post-sleep increase in dolorimeter scores and a subjective increase in pain and stiffness. Seven of the 10 patients had NREM stages 2, 3, and 4 contaminated by an intercurrent alpha rhythm. The three patients without this pattern had no stage 4 sleep and little or no stage 3 sleep.

The authors suggested a relationship between disturbed SWS and the musculoskeletal pain, and performed further studies to substantiate this. Six healthy volunteers, ages nineteen to twenty-four years, were studied during baseline sleep, stage 4 sleep deprivation, and recovery. Subjects reported significantly increased muscle pain and stiffness, had increased dolorimeter scores, and showed the alpha-delta NREM disturbance after stage 4 deprivation. In yet another study (Moldofsky & Scarisbrick, 1976), seven healthy volunteers were deprived of REM sleep and showed no significant increase in musculoskeletal symptoms, although some did report tiredness and irritability. And finally, six patients with rheumatoid arthritis were studied and, like those with fibrositis syndrome, had an alpha-NREM sleep disturbance and increased pain and stiffness with decreased grip strength post-sleep (Moldofsky, Lue, Peacock, & Smythe, 1977). The authors suggest that a disturbance of NREM sleep may lead to emergence of certain musculoskeletal symptoms and may be the result of a disturbance in serotonin metabolism. This is an interesting suggestion and one that merits further investigation.

SLEEP AND INFECTIONS/FEVER

Probably everyone has experienced disturbed sleep during an acute viral or bacterial illness. Perhaps because it's "common sense" that a person doesn't sleep well during a gastroenteritis or respiratory infection and because the sleep disturbance is usually self-limited, almost no study has been done on the subject.

Karacan, Wolff, Williams, Hursch, and Webb (1968) studied the effects of a pyrogen (etiocholanolone) on sleep in 11 healthy male medical students. The mean temerature among the subjects reached the highest level of 38.9°C at 1 a.m. and was 37.4°C by awakening. Subjects with fever had significantly more awakenings, reduced amounts of REM sleep, reduced stage 4 sleep in the first third of the night, and increased stage 4 sleep in the last third of the night. Overall percentage of stage 4 sleep was decreased. Latency to sleep onset, latency to REM sleep, and amount of stage 0 sleep were all significantly increased. The frequency and duration of awakenings increased as temperature increased. One subject who did not develop an increase in temperature and one who was given aspirin did not have increased temperature and did not have any changes in sleep patterns. Thus, available data in humans support the conventional wisdom that fever does cause restless, disturbed sleep. The etiology of this effect is unknown.

Sleep can become of paramount importance in some infectious diseases, particularly those of the respiratory tract. In severe pneumonia, for example, the already compromised respiratory function is decreased by sleep (see section on sleep and respiratory function). This can lead to hypoxia and death. In infants nasopharyngitis has been statistically implicated in sudden infant death syndrome sleep apnea (Steinschneider, 1975), although polysomnography was not done.

SLEEP AND ENDOCRINOPATHIES

There have been a number of animal and human studies of endocrine function in sleep but few of sleep in endocrine disorders. In normals several patterns of endocrine release in sleep have been documented: (1) growth hormone peaks early in the night during NREM sleep, particularly SWS (Karacan, Rosenbloom, et al., 1973; Parker, Rossman, et al., 1980); (2) if sleep is delayed or advanced, there is a corresponding shift in the time of secretion of growth hormone; (3) growth hormone release and sleep may be dissociated in certain patient populations, such as narcoleptics, schizophrenics, patients with Cushing's syndrome, depressed patients (Orem & Keeling, 1980); (4) prolactin secretion peaks during late sleep (Parker, Rossman, et al., 1980); (5) in puberty, luteinizing hormone (LH) secretion, and thus testosterone levels in males, are directly related to sleep; disturbed sleep results in disturbed LH patterns; and (6) thyroid-stimulating hormone peaks in the evening and is inhibited by sleep (Parker, Pekary, & Hershman 1976).

Diabetes Mellitus

There have been no notable differences found in the sleep of diabetic outpatients and healthy control subjects (Karacan, Salis, et al., 1978).

Hypothyroidism

Hypothyroid patients are often noted to be lethargic or somnolent. However, nocturnal EEG studies of seven hypothyroid adults revealed no difference from normals' TST, sleep-onset latency, percentage of REM sleep, and number and intervals of REM periods. SWS was decreased and stage 2 sleep increased. All of the four of the seven who were restudied after hormone treatment had a normalization of SWS (Kales, Heuser, et al., 1967).

Five hypothyroid infants and children aged four weeks and three years had delayed development of sleep spindles. The development of sleep spindles is a sign of neurophysiological maturation. After thyroid hormone therapy, spindling increased in the three- to eight-month-old infants but not in the older child (Schultz, Schulte, Akiyama, & Parmelee, 1968). These findings are consistent with the fact that unless hypothyroid infants are treated early, permanent brain dysfunction results.

Hyperthyroidism

Hyperthyroid patients often complain of insomnia, but there are conflicting objective reports of the effects of hyperthyroidism on sleep. Passouant, Passouant-Fontaine, and Cadilhac (1966) found decreased TST and percentage of SWS and increased sleep onset latency compared with normals. Dunleavy and Oswald (1972) reported increased percentages of time spent in SWS, which gradually reverted to normal after treatment.

Hyperparathyroidism

We know of only two patients with this disorder who have been studied polysomnographically (Foster et al., 1977). They had mild to moderate hypercalcemia and showed absence of SWS, decreased sleep efficiency, decreased REM-onset latency, and increased REM density and incidence of rapid eye movements in stage 2 sleep. These patients also suffered depression, however, which confuses the interpretation of the sleep disturbances.

Endocrinopathy and Sleep Apnea

There are at least two case reports of sleep apnea in patients with endocrinopathy; i.e., hypothyroidism (Yamamoto, Hirose, & Miyoshi, 1977) and acromegaly (Mezon, West, MacLean, & Kryger, 1980). Both patients had macroglossia and upper airway obstructive sleep apnea.

SLEEP AND OBESITY, FASTING, AND ANOREXIA NERVOSA

Associations of sleep changes and changes in food intake and body weight have been noted for a number of years; for example, in the Klein-Levin syndrome of hypersomnia and megaphagia and in lesions of the ventromedial nucleus of the hypothalamus. Furthermore, in depressive states insomnia and weight loss are often coupled.

We studied 11 healthy medical students during baseline and up to 67 h of fasting (Karacan, Rosenbloom, et al., 1973). Thirty to 37 h of fasting produced no significant changes in EEG sleep patterns. However, 60 to 67 h of fasting produced a significant increase in stage 4 sleep, a compensatory decrease in stage 2 sleep, and a decrease in the number of REM periods. There were no other significant changes in sleep patterns. The decrease in the number of REM periods in fasting may be consistent with a current concept that protein synthesis is important in the regulation of REM sleep, but the etiology of the decrease is unknown.

Lacey, Crisp, Kalucy, Hartmann, and Chen (1975) studied polysomnographically 10 patients with anorexia nervosa at baseline low weight and during hospitalization with weight gain. SWS initially increased, and there were significant increases in total sleep and REM sleep toward normal.

Crisp, Stonehill, Fenton, and Fenwick (1973) studied five obese females hospitalized and consuming a 500-calorie diet. Sleep evaluation was done by questionnaire and intermittent sleep EEG studies. Total sleep decreased as the patients' weights decreased. There were relative increases in stage 2 sleep and decreases in stage 4 sleep over the 4-month hospital stay. Other researchers found a significant fall in REM sleep with acute starvation (McFadyen, Oswald, & Lewis, 1973) and a direct correlation between body weight and percentage of total sleep in REM sleep (Adam, 1977).

Obesity, of course, can be related to other disorders that can disturb sleep, such as sleep apnea, cardiovascular disorders, and endocrinopathy, which are discussed elsewhere.

DERMATOLOGIC PROBLEMS AND SLEEP

There have been at least three studies of pruritic dermatologic conditons and sleep. Sleep was clearly disturbed in each of the patient populations. Savin, Paterson, and Oswald (1973) and Savin, Paterson, Oswald, and Adam (1975) performed polysomnography on 4 and 15 patients, respectively, with itchy skin diseases. Scratching occurred during all stages of sleep. Scratching was most frequent in stage 1. The frequency decreased through stages 2, 3, and 4. Statistically significant decreases were observed when LS (stages 1 and 2) was compared to SWS (stages 3 and 4). The frequency of scratching in REM sleep was comparable to that in stage 2, and scratching while awake but in bed and in stage 1 were about equally frequent. The mean duration of scratching bouts was about 10 seconds for all sleep stages and 15 seconds for waking.

Brown and Kalucy (1975) studied four adults with pruritic skin conditioins in an effort to discover psychological factors and personality styles related to nighttime scratching. The four patients were referred by dermatologists to the authors for psychological studies because of "marked nighttime scratching." This method of referral was not random and may have biased the sample toward increased psychopathology, in that the patients chosen by the dermatologists for sleep and psychiatric evaluation may have been those who seemed more emotionally disturbed or complained more of poor sleep. Scratching occurred in all sleep stages and was more in the first half of the night. Although the actual data and the control data were not provided, the authors generalized that the patients showed more nocturnal movements, longer sleep-onset latency, and less SWS than expected in normal subjects. Personality and hostility inventories showed the patients "tended to be introverted neurotics with a high level of aggression directed mainly inwards."

SLEEP AND HEMATOLOGIC DISORDERS

Paroxysmal nocturnal hemoglobinuria (PNH) is a disorder exacerbated by sleep. In PNH, hemolysis is increased during sleep, regardless of time of day of the sleep. Hansen (1968) monitored the plasma hemoglobin (Hgb) of seven patients over a 24-h period without the benefit of polysomnography. Five patients had increased plasma Hgb that was maximal at about midnight and/or 4 a.m. during sleep and that rapidly decreased on awakening. Increased plasma Hgb indicates increased hemolysis. One patient with "mild PNH" showed no significant diurnal change, and one, whose past clinical history was more ambiguous (causing the author to question the PNH diagnosis), had decreased plasma Hgb while asleep. All of four patients monitored during daytime sleep had increased plasma Hgb. The mechanism of this phenomenon is unknown but may be related to sluggish circulation in the spleen, decreased cortisol, or decreased blood pH secondary to increased P_{CO2} in sleep.

There is some evidence that polycythemia and sleep may be mutually exacerbating conditions. We know of one case report of a patient with polycythemia rubra vera who suffered 52 episodes of central sleep apnea with multiple microarousals when his packed cell volume (PCV) was 65 percent; after phlebotomy to a PCV of 49 percent the apnea disappeared (Neil, Reynolds, Spiker, & Kupfer, 1980). This suggests the disordered sleep was caused by increased PCV. This hypothesis also is supported by Stradling and Lane (1980), who reported one case with chronic obstructive pulmonary disease (COPD) and secondary polycy-

themia who had improved nocturnal hypoxia after phlebotomy. Other authors, with larger samples, believe the converse,
that the sleep hypoxia due to sleep apnea or lung disease is the
cause of increased polycythemia (Douglas et al., 1979; Kryger
et al., 1978). These are not, of course, mutually exclusive hy-
potheses.

SLEEP AND OPHTHALMOLOGIC DISORDERS

Corneal Erosions

Sturrock (1976) examined 102 patients believed to have
suffered corneal exposure during sleep due to incomplete closure of eyelids. The incidence was highest in the third decade
and declined with increasing age. Slightly less than one-half of
the patients had suffered previous episodes. By history, the only
identified possible etiologic factor was alcohol intake before
bedtime, which was admitted by 51 percent of the patients.

Blindness

A pilot survey of "the blind community" in California was
done by Miles and Wilson (1977). Fifty questionnaires were returned by partially to totally blind persons. Seventy-six percent
complained of a sleep disturbance, severe enough to interfere
with work in 36 percent and to require medication in 24 percent. Of course, the sample may have been biased by those returning the questionnaires having more problems with sleep.

SLEEP AND DEAFNESS

To the casual observer, sleep in deaf people is no different from that in normals (Robinson & Dawson, 1975). In fact,
one might expect sleep to be less fragmented or disturbed because of the decreased sensitivity to arousing noises. Four young
adult congenitally deaf males monitored polysomnographically

for 5 consecutive nights were found to have significantly less NREM sleep and SWS and spent more time awake than normal controls (Robinson & Dawson, 1975). Further studies with larger samples are necessary before any conclusions about sleep in deaf persons can be drawn.

CONCLUSION

Basic sleep physiology and sleep in a variety of medical and surgical conditions have been reviewed in this chapter. Sleep in some of these conditions has been systematically studied; in others only case reports are available. All disease states in which systematic sleep studies are available were reviewed. However, it is clear that much research remains to be done; the dearth of information can be explained in part by ethical and methodological considerations. Central questions left for future research include whether sleep is important in recovery from illnesses, whether disturbed sleep exacerbates certain disease states or contributes to developing disease processes, and how sleep-induced changes in illnesses (e.g., PNH, nocturnal asthma, nocturnal angina, and others) are mediated. Answers to these questions also will add to our understanding of the function of sleep and provide a basis for rational treatments of sleep-related disorders.

REFERENCES

Adam, K. (1977). Body weight correlates with REM sleep. *British Journal of medicine, 1*(6064), 813–814.

Bateman, J. R. M., Clarke, S. W., Pavia, D., & Sheahan, N. F. (1978). Reduction of clearance secretions from the human lung during sleep. *Journal of Physiology, 284,* 55–57.

Bergonzi, P., Bianco, A., Mazza, S., & Mennuni, G. (1978). Night sleep organization in patients with severe hepatic failure: Its modifications after L-dopa treatment. *European Neurology, 17*(5), 271–275.

Billiard, M., Guilleminault, C., & Dement, W. C. (1975). A menstruation-linked periodic hypersomnia. *Neurology, 25,* 436–443.

Bonhuye, A. (1963). Effect of posture on experimental asthma in man. *American Journal of Medicine, 34,* 470–476.

Booth, D. J., Kemmerer, W. G., & Skinner, D. B. (1968). Acid clearing from the distal esophagus. *Archives of Surgery, 96,* 731–734.

Broughton, R., & Baron, R. (1973). Sleep of acute coronary patients in an open ward type intensive care unit. *Sleep Research, 2,* 144.

Brown, D. C., & Kalucy, R. S. (1975). Correlation of neurophysiological and personality data in sleep scratching. *Proceedings of the Royal Medical Society, 68,* 530–532.

Clark, T. J. H., & Hetzel, M. R. (1977). Diurnal variation of asthma. *British Journal of Diseases of the Chest, 71,* 87–92.

Coccagna, G., Mantovani, M., Brignani, F., Manzini, A., & Lugaresi, E. (1971). Laboratory note: Arterial pressure changes during spontaneous sleep in man. *Electroencephalography and Clinical Neurophysiology, 31,* 277–281.

Condie, R. (1979). Chlormezanone in the treatment of insomnia due to rheumatic stiffness. *Current Medical Research and Opinion, 6*(3), 217–220.

Criep, L. H. (1969). *Clinical immunology and allergy,* 2d ed. New York: Grune & Stratton.

Crisp, A. H., Stonehill, E., Fenton, G. W., Fenwick, P. B. C. (1973). Sleep patterns in obese patients during weight reduction. *Psychotherapy and Psychosomatics, 22,* 159–165.

DeMeester, T. R., & Johnson, L. F. (1975). Position of the esophageal sphincter and its relationship to reflux. *Surgical Forum, 26,* 364–366.

de Vries, K., Goei, J. T., Booy-Noord, H., & Orie, N. G. M. (1962). Changes during 24 hours in the lung function and histamine hyperactivity of the bronchial tree in asthmatic and bronchitic patients. *International Archives of Allergy and Applied Immunology, 20,* 93–101.

Dlin, B. M., Rosen, H., Dickstein, K., Lyons, J. W., & Fischer, H. K. (1971). The problems of sleep and rest in the intensive care unit. *Psychosomatics, 12,* 155–163.

Douglas, N. J., Caverly, P. M. A., Leggett, R. J. E., Brash, H. M., Flenley, D. C., & Brezinova, V. (1979). Transient hypoxaemia during sleep in chronic bronchitis and emphysema. *Lancet, 1,* 1–4.

Dragstedt, L. R. (1959). Causes of peptic ulcer. *Journal of the American Medical Association, 169,* 203–209.

Dunleavy, D. L. F., & Oswald, I. (1972). Sleep and thyrotoxicosis. *Sleep Research, 1,* 385.

Elwell, E. L., Frankel, B. L., & Snyder, F. (1974). A polygraphic sleep study of five cardiotomy patients. *Sleep Research, 3,* 133.

Fink, B. R. (1961). Influence of cerebral activity in wakefulness on regulation of breathing. *Journal of Applied Physiology, 16,* 15–20.

Flick, M. R., & Block, A. J. (1979). Nocturnal vs. diurnal cardiac arrythmias in patients with chronic obstructive pulmonary disease. *Chest, 75,* 8–11.

Foster, F. G., Holzer, B., Spiker, D. G., Love, D., Coble, P., & Kupfer, D. J. (1977). Stones, bones, moans, and groans: Mood and sleep in primary hyperparathyroidism. *Sleep Research, 6,* 188.

Glenn, W. W., Holcomb, W. G., Shaw, R. K., Hogan, J. F., & Halschuh, K. R. (1976). Long term ventilatory support by diaphragm pacing in quadriplegia. *Annals of Surgery, 183,* 566–577.

Guazzi, M., Bacelli, G., & Zanchetti, A. (1968). Reflex chemoceptive regulation of arterial pressure during natural sleep in the cat. *American Journal of Physiology, 214,* 969–978.

Guazzi, M., & Zanchetti, A. (1965). Carotid sinus and aortic reflexes in the regulation of circulation during sleep. *Science, 148,* 397–399.

Guilleminault, C., & Dement, W. C. (1978). Sleep apnea syndromes and related disorders. In R. L. Williams & I. Karacan (Eds.), *Sleep disorders: Diagnoses and treatment.* (pp. 9–28) New York: John Wiley.

Gunderson, C. H., Dunne, P. B., & Feyer, T. L. (1973). Sleep deprivation and seizures. *Neurology, 23,* 678–686.

Hansen, N. E. (1968). Sleep related plasma haemoglobin levels in paroxysmal nocturnal haemoglobuinuria. *Acta Medica Scandinavica, 184,* 547–549.

Hartmann, E. L. (1966). The D-state (dreaming sleep) and the menstrual cycle. *Recent Advances in Biological Psychiatry, 8,* 34–35.

Hetzel, M. R., & Clark, T. J. H. (1979). Does sleep cause nocturnal asthma? *Thorax, 34,* 749–754.

Johnson, L. F. (1969). Psychological and physiological changes following total sleep deprivation. In A. Kales (Ed.), *Sleep: Physiology and pathology.* (pp. 43–59) Philadelphia: J. B. Lippincott.

Johnson, L. F., & DeMeester, T. R. (1974). Twenty-four hour pH monitoring of the distal esophagus: A quantitative measure of the gastroesophageal reflux. *American Journal of Gastroenterology, 62,* 325–332.

Johnson, L. F., DeMeester, T. R., & Haggitt, R. C. (1978). Esophageal epithelial response to gastroesophageal reflux: A quantitative study. *American Journal of Digestive Diseases, 23,* 458–459.

Kales, A., Beall, G. N., Bajor, G. F., Jacobson, A., & Kales, J. (1968). Sleep studies in asthmatic adults: Relationships of attacks to sleep stage and time of night. *Journal of Allergy, 41,* 164–173.

Kales, A., Heuser, G., Jacobson, A., Kales, J. D., Hanley, J., Zweizig, J. R., & Paulson, M. J. (1967). All-night sleep studies in hypothyroid patients, before and after treatment. *Journal of Clinical Endocrinology, 27,* 1593–1599.

Kales, A., Kales, J. D., & Sly, R. M. (1973). Sleep patterns of asthmatic children: All-night electroencephalographic studies. *Journal of Allergy, 46,* 300–308.

Karacan, I., Green, J. R., Taylor, W. J., Williams, J. C., Eliot, R. S., Thornby, J. I., Salis, P. J., & Williams, R. L. (1973). Sleep characteristics of acute myocardial infarct patients in an ICU unit. *Sleep Research, 2,* 159.

Karacan, I., Guinn, G., Mathur, V., Anch, M., McCoy, G., Freeborg, G., Ware, C., & Williams, R. L. (1977). The incidence of premature ventricular contractions during sleep in patients with coronary artery disease. *Sleep Research, 6,* 189.

Karacan, I., Rosenbloom, A. L., Londono, J. H., Salis, P. J., Thornby, J. I., & Williams, R. L. (1973). The effect of acute fasting on sleep and the sleep-growth hormone response. *Psychosomatics, 14,* 33–37.

Karacan, I., Salis, P. J., Ware, J. C., Dervent, B., Williams, R. L., Scott, F. B., Attia, S. L., & Beutler, L. (1978). Nocturnal penile tumescence and diagnosis in diabetic impotence. *American Journal of Psychiatry, 135,* 191–197.

Karacan, I., & Williams, R. L. (1970). Current advances in theory and practice relating to postpartum syndrome. *Psychiatry in Medicine, 1,* 307–328.

Karacan, I., Williams, R. L., Bose, J., Hursch, C. J., & Warson, S. R. (1972). Insomnia in hemodialytic and kidney transplant patients. *Psychophysiology, 9,* 137.

Karacan, I., Williams, R. L., & Taylor, W. J. (1969). Sleep characteristics of patients with angina pectoris. *Psychosomatics, 10,* 280–284.

Karacan, I., Wolff, S. M., Williams, R. L., Hursch, C. J., & Webb, W. B. (1968). The effects of fever on sleep and dream patterns. *Psychosomatics, 9,* 331–339.

Khatri, I. M., & Freis, E. D. (1967). Hemodynamic changes during sleep. *Journal of Applied Physiology, 22,* 868–873.

Koo, K. W., Sax, D. S., & Snider, G. L. (1975). Arterial blood gases and pH during sleep in chronic obstructive pulmonary disease. *American Journal of Medicine, 58,* 663–670.

Kryger, M., Glas, R., Jackson, D., McCullough, R. E., Scoggin, C., Grover, R. F., & Weil, J. V. (1978). Impaired oxygenation during sleep in excessive polycythemia of high altitude: Improvement with respiratory stimulation. *Sleep, 1,* 3–17.

Kukorelli, T., & Juhasz, G. (1977). Sleep induced by intestinal stimulation in cats. *Physiology and Behavior, 19,* 355–358.

Kukorelli, T., & Juhasz, G. (1978). Electroencephalographic synchronization induced by stimulation of small intestine and splanchnic nerve in cats. *Electroencephalography and Clinical Neurophysiology, 41,* 491–500.

Lacey, J. H., Crisp, A. H., Kalucy, R. S., Hartmann, M. K., & Chen, C. N. (1975). Weight gain and the sleeping electroencephalogram: Study of 10 patients with anorexia nervosa. *British Journal of Medicine, 4,* 556–558.

Levy, A. M., Camm, A. J., & Keane, J. P. (1977). Multiple arrhythmias detected during nocturnal monitoring in patients with congenital complete heart block. *Circulation, 55,* 247–253.

Lichter, I., & Muir, R. C. (1975). The pattern of swallowing during sleep. *Electroencephalography and Clinical Neurophysiology, 38,* 427–432.

Lown, B., Tykocinski, M., Garfein, A., & Brooks, P. (1973). Sleep and ventricular beats. *Circulation, 51,* 691–701.

MacWilliams, J. A. (1923). Blood pressure and heart action in sleep and dreams: Their relation to hemorrhages, angina and sudden death. *British Journal of Medicine, 22,* 1196–1200.

Mancia, G., Bacelli, G., Adams, D. B., & Zanchetti, A. (1971). Vasomotor regulation during sleep in the cat. *American Journal of Physiology, 220,* 1086–1093.

Mandell, A. J., Chaffey, B., Brill, P., Mandell, M. P., Rodnick, J., Rubin, R. T., & Sheff, R. (1966). Dreaming sleep in men: Changes in urine volume and osmolality. *Science, 151,* 1558–1560.

McFadden, E. H., & Giblin, E. C. (1971). Sleep deprivation in patients having open heart surgery. *Nursing Research, 2,* 249–254.

McFadyen, U. M., Oswald, I., & Lewis, S. A. (1973). Starvation and human slow-wave sleep. *Applied Physiology, 35,* 391–394.

Mezon, B. L., West, P., Israels, J., & Kryger, M. (1980). Sleep breathing abnormalities in kyphoscoliosis. *American Review of Respiratory Disorders, 122,* 617–621.

Mezon, B. J., West, P., Maclean, J. P., & Kryger, M. H. (1980). Sleep apnea in acromegaly. *American Journal of Medicine, 69,* 615–618.

Miles, L. E., & Wilson, M. P. (1977). High incidence of cyclic sleep-wake disorders in the blind. *Sleep Research, 6,* 192.

Miller, J. C., & Helander, M. (1979). The 24-hour cycle and the nocturnal depression of human cardiac output. *Aviation Space and Environmental Medicine, 50,* 1139–1144.

Moldofsky, H., Lue, F., Peacock, J., & Smythe, H. (1977). Alpha non-REM sleep and musculoskeletal symptoms in rheumatoid arthritis. *Sleep Research, 6,* 193.

Moldofsky, H., Scarisbrick, P., England, R., & Smythe, H. (1975). Musculoskeletal symptoms and non-REM sleep disturbance in patients with fibrositis syndrome and healthy subjects. *Psychosomatic Medicine, 37,* 341–351.

Moldofsky, H., & Scarisbrick, P. (1976). Induction of neurasthenic musculoskeletal pain syndrome by selective sleep stage deprivation. *Psychosomatic Medicine, 38,* 35–44.

Monti, J. M., Folle, L. E., Peluffo, C., Artucio, R., Ortiz, A., Sevrini, O., & Dighiero, J. (1975). The incidence of premature contractions in coronary patients during the sleep-wake cycle. *Cardiology, 60,* 257–264.

Mullen, P. E., James, V. H., Lightman, S. L., Linsell, C., & Peart, W. S. (1980). A relationship between plasma renin activity and rapid eye movement phase of sleep in man. *Endocrinology and Metabolism, 50,* 466–469.

Neil, J. F., Reynolds, C. F., 3rd, Spiker, D. G., & Kupfer, D. J. (1980). Polycythaemia and central sleep apnea. *British Medical Journal, 280*(6206), 1.

Nichols, C., Tyler, F. H. (1967). Diurnal variation in adrenal cortical function. *Annual Review of Medicine, 18,* 313–324.

Nowlin, J. B., Troyer, W. G., Collins, W. S., Silverman, G., Nichols, C. R., McIntosh, H. D., Estes, E. H., & Bogdonoff, M. D. (1965). The association of nocturnal angina pectoris with dreaming. *Annals of Internal Medicine, 63,* 1040–1046.

Orem, J., & Keeling, J. (1980). Appendix: A compendium of physiology in sleep. In J. Orem & C. D. Barnes (Eds.), *Physiology in sleep.* New York: Academic Press.

Orr, W. C., Hall, W. H., & Stahl, M. L., Durkin, M. G., & Whitsett, T. L. (1976). Sleep patterns and gastric acid secretion in duodenal ulcer disease. *Archives of Internal Medicine, 136,* 655–660.

Orr, W. C., Langevin, E., & Stahl, M. L. (1977). Cardiac arrhythmias during sleep in the prolapsed mitral valve syndrome. *Sleep Research, 6,* 196.

Orr, W. C., & Stahl, M. L. (1977). Sleep disturbance after open heart surgery. *American Journal of Cardiology, 39,* 196–201.

Parker, D. C., Pekary, A. E., & Hershman, J. M. (1976). Effects of normal and reversed sleep-wake cycles upon nyctohemeral rhythmicity of plasma thyrotropin: Evidence suggestive of an inhibitory influence in sleep. *Journal of Clinical Endocrinology and Metabolism, 43,* 318–329.

Parker, D. C., Rossman, L. G., Kripke, D. F., Hershman, J. M., Gibson, W., Davis, C., Wilson, K., & Pekary, E. (1980). Endocrine rhythms across sleep-wake cycles in normal young men under basal state conditions. In J. Orem & C. D. Barnes (Eds.), *Physiology in sleep.* New York: Academic Press.

Passouant, P., Cadilhac, J., Baldy-Moulinier, M., & Mion, C. (1970). Etude du sommeil nocturne chez des uremiques chroniques soumis à une épuration extrarenale. *Electroencephalography and Clinical Neurophysiology, 2,* 441–449.

Passouant, P., Passouant-Fontaine, T., & Cadilhac, J. (1966). L'influence de l'hyperthyroidie sur le sommeil. Etude clinique et experimentale. *Revue Neurologique, 115,* 353–366.

Ravenscroft, K., & Hartmann, E. (1968). The temporal correlation of nocturnal asthmatic attacks and the D-state. *Psychophysiology, 4,* 396–397.

Regestein, Q. R., DeSilva, R. A., & Lown, B. (1981). Cardiac ventricular ectopic activity increases during REM sleep. *Sleep Research, 10,* 58.

Robinson, L. D., & Dawson, S. D. (1975). EEG and REM sleep studies in deaf people. *American Annals of the Deaf, 120,* 387–390.

Rosenblatt, G., Hartmann, E., & Azillig, G. R. (1973). Cardiac irritability during sleep and dreaming. *Journal of Psychosomatic Research, 17,* 129–134.

Rubin, R. T. (1980). Hormonal regulation of renal function during sleep. In J. Orem & C. D. Barnes (Eds.), *Physiology in sleep*. New York: Academic Press.

Sassin, J. F. (1970). Neurological findings following short-term sleep deprivation. *Archives of Neurology, 22*, 54–56.

Savin, J. A., Paterson, W. D., & Oswald, I. (1973). Scratching during sleep. *Lancet, 2*, 296–297.

Savin, J. A., Paterson, W. D., Oswald, I., & Adam, K. (1975). Further studies of scratching during sleep. *British Journal of Dermatology, 93*, 297–302.

Schultz, M. A., Shulte, F. J., Akiyama, Y., Parmelee, A. H. (1968). Development of electroencephalographic sleep phenomena in hypothyroid infants. *Electroencephalography and Clinical Neurophysiology, 25*, 351–358.

Smith, R., Johnson, L., Rothfeld, D., Zir, L., & Tharp, B. (1972). Sleep and cardiac arrhythmias. *Archives of Internal Medicine, 130*, 342–349.

Soutar, C. A., Carruthers, M., & Pickering, C. A. (1977). Nocturnal asthma and urinary adrenaline and noradrenaline excretion. *Thorax, 32*, 677–683.

Stacher, G., Presslich, B., & Starker, H. (1975). Gastric acid secretion and sleep stages during natural night sleep. *Gastroenterology, 68*, 1449–1455.

Steinschneider, A. (1975). Nasopharyngitis and prolonged sleep apnea. *Pediatrics, 56*, 967–971.

Stern, S., & Tzivoni, D. (1973). Dynamic changes in the ST-T segment during sleep in ischemic heart disease. *American Journal of Cardiology, 23*, 17–20.

Stradling, J. R., & Lane, D. J. (1980). Polycythemia vera and central sleep apnea. *British Medical Journal, 280*(6211), 404.

Sturrock, G. O. (1976). Nocturnal lagophthalmos and recurrent erosion. *British Journal of Opthalmalogy, 60*, 97–103.

Sullivan, C. E. (1980). Breathing in sleep. In J. Orem & C. D. Barnes (Eds.), *Physiology in sleep*. New York: Academic Press.

Trask, C. H., & Cree, E. M. (1962). Oximeter studies on patients with chronic obstructive emphysema, awake and during sleep. *New England Journal of Medicine, 266*, 639–642.

Turner-Warwick, M. (1977). On observing patterns of airflow obstruction in chronic asthma. *British Journal of Diseases of the Chest, 71*, 73–85.

Vogel, J. H. K., Kelminson, L. L., & Cotton, E. K. (1967). Pulmonary hypertension during sleep. *American Journal of Diseases of Children,* *113,* 576–580.

Yamamoto, T., Hirose, N., & Miyoshi, K. (1977). Polygraphic study of periodic breathing and hypersomnolence in a patient with severe hypothyroidism. *European Neurology, 15*(4), 188–193.

Chapter 6

THE DIAGNOSIS, ONTOGENESIS, AND MANAGEMENT OF HYPOCHONDRIASIS*

James J. Strain

Hypochondriasis was first described as a disease in 350 B.C. by Diocles, who associated the disorder with digestive organs. It has occupied the attention of physicians throughout the centuries and was not lost sight of in the third and latest edition of the *Diagnostic and Statistical Manual of Mental Disorders* (DSM III) (1980), despite the debate that continues as to whether it is a primary or secondary phenomenon. In fact, it was placed in the category of the somatoform disorders as a state disturbance (Axis I). This phenomenological approach sidesteps the issue of etiology altogether.

---

*Many of the formulations presented in this chapter have been articulated in N. Altman (1975); Ladde (1966) in his monograph on the hypochondriacal syndrome presents a historical perspective of the term and the disease; Kenyan (1976) provides a review and historical background.

This work has been supported by NIMH Training Grant MH 16438–01 and the Green Foundation.

In the DSM III hypochondriasis is listed as one of the five somatoform disorders: (1) somatization disorder (Briquet's syndrome), (2) conversion reaction, (3) psychogenic pain, (4) hypochondriasis, (5) atypical somatoform disorder.

Hypochondriasis in DSM III (1980) has been described as having at least four features:

1. The predominant disturbance is an unrealistic interpretation of physical signs or sensations as abnormal, leading to preoccupation with the fear or belief of having a serious disease.

2. Thorough physical evaluation does not support the diagnosis of any physical disorder that can account for the physical signs or sensations or for the individual's unrealistic interpretation of them.

3. The unrealistic fear or belief of having a disease persists despite medical reassurance and causes impairment in social or occupational functioning.

4. The disturbance is not due to any other mental disorder such as schizophrenia, affective disorder, or somatoform disorder.

But hypochondriasis remains a diagnostic dilemma, and the correct diagnosis of its etiology is essential for an appropriate intervention. Hypochondriasis and the other somatoform disorders highlight the problem of dissociating a state disturbance (Axis I) from a personality disorder (Axis II). For example, the narcissistic and borderline personality disorders are frequently characterized by hypochondriacal behavior that can mimic a state disturbance at times of stress, conflict, and regression (Kernberg, 1975; Kohut, 1964). Both Lipsitt (1970) and Altman (1975) describe the masochistic personality disorder that invariably is present in the patient who manifests severe clinical hypochondriasis. Is hypochondriasis a personality disorder with pronounced somatic features and symptoms?

In fact, with greater attention to the possible presence of other psychiatric diseases and personality disorders giving rise to somatic preoccupation and the conviction of illness out of keeping with reality, more and more "secondary" hypochondriasis would be observed. Consequently, fewer of the residual patient group would remain in the category of "true" (or primary) hypochondriasis. From his investigation of a substantial number of patients, Kenyan (1964), in contrast to many other investigators, concluded that hypochondriasis is always part of another condition, usually a depressive illness. Similarly, when a group of hypochondriacal patients in a general hospital were studied, using the Missouri Mental State Examination, the majority did have other psychiatric disorders (Table 6-1).

Hypochondriasis also may be secondary to depressive disorders, organic brain syndromes, unresolved grief, psychophysiologic disorders, malingering, and obsessional neuroses.*

The importance of differential diagnosis cannot be overestimated, therefore, as exemplified by the large number of psychiatric disorders of which it may be a symptom. Hypochondriasis is a secondary phenomenon in these diagnostic groups and is treated by addressing the primary disorder, e.g., depression, schizophrenia, conversion reactions, somatoform disorders.

Primary hypochondriasis is not associated with another psychiatric reaction and is characterized by the following: (1) functional disorder; (2) character problem; (3) lifelong style of behavior; (4) product of a fixation or a regression; (5) possible worsening with stress.

Turnbull (1974) described those individuals who temporarily under stress experience a conviction of illness and transient somatic symptoms of psychogenic origin as "temporary hypochondriasis." Ehrlich (1980) described this syndrome as reactive hypochondriasis versus essential. It also has been labeled the "medical student syndrome." Mechanic (1973) reports that three of four people have symptoms in any given

---

*Pilowsky (1970) previously described primary and secondary hypochondriasis. Munro (1978) described the successful treatment with pimozide of monosymptomatic hypochondriacal psychosis manifesting as delusions of parasitosis. Although the drug did not effect a cure, it resulted in a remission of symptoms.

Table 6-1. Presence of Hypochondriacal Symptoms in
Consultation/Psych-Med Unit Patients*

Ward	Age	Sex	Severity of Psychiatric Disorder	DSM III Axis I
10	35	F	moderate	300.81 Somatization disorder
183	43	M	mild	300.11 Conversion disorder
3	69	F	severe	300.81 Somatization disorder
100	48	F	mild	300.40 Dysthymic disorder
26	67	F	mild	29622 Major affective disorder
201	45	M	mild	297.10 Paranoia
42	74	F	mild	296.50 Bipolar disorder
16	33	F	severe	295.30 Schizophrenic disorder, paranoid type
104	41	F	mild	300.11 Conversion disorder
100	27	F	mild	V7109 No diagnosis
100	71	F	mild	296.34 Major affective disorder
42	69	F	severe	296.20 Major affective disorder
42	67	M	moderate	296.20 Major affective disorder
42	21	M	severe	300.16 Factitious disorder
25	75	F	mild	309.00 Adjustment disorder with depressed mood

*Hypochondriacal symptoms reflected on the Missouri Mental Status Examination in a 4-month consultation population at Mt. Sinai Hospital, New York.

month for which they take some definable action, such as use of medication, bed rest, consulting a physician, and limiting activity.

PSEUDOHYPOCHONDRIASIS OF THE AGED

Recent gerontological studies challenge the notion that a large proportion of the aged suffer from hypochondriasis (Busse, 1982; Palmore, 1970; Strain, 1978). It is my impression that many elderly patients who manifest clinical features of hypochondriasis should be diagnosed as suffering from "pseudohypochondriasis."

The most prominent characteristic of the hypochondriac is a long-standing preoccupation with bodily concerns, accompanied by vague, shifting somatic complaints that are markedly exaggerated in relation to physical findings. A similar excessive concern with bodily function of more recent onset might be regarded as normal in the aged. Given the biological changes inherent in the aging process, the frequent expression of vague somatic complaints by elderly patients does not have the same prognostic implications.

In both hypochondriasis and pseudohypochondriasis the preoccupation with bodily function replaces the individual's interest in external objects. Both the hypochondriac and the pseudohypochondriac attempt, on the basis of illness and suffering, to establish a regressive relationship with the physician, who on another level is perceived as a social contact. Patients in both groups have a paucity of social relationships. However, the elderly individual's social isolation is usually age-related; in the case of the true hypochondriac, the lack of viable social relationships is a consequence of lifelong aberrant behavior.

The fact that the hypochondriac's somatic complaints are not significantly relieved by traditional medical treatment stems from his/her need to be sick in order to have prolonged and repeated medical contact. To this end, the hypochondriac incriminates "innocent" organs and willingly submits to and even demands life-threatening procedures. When the clinical workup shows no organic pathology to account for the type or degree of symptomatology, the hypochondriacal patient responds to this reassurance with anger and an increase of complaints, insisting on further procedures. In contrast, the pseudohypochondriac's response to a favorable diagnosis is one of relief. He/she derives no comfort from the prospect of undergoing complex, costly, and often uncomfortable diagnostic and therapeutic procedures.

Finally, the true hypochondriac tends in the medical setting to manifest persecutory trends, that is, to level accusations of neglect, rejection, and incompetence against the physician. Such behavior is not characteristic of the aged pseudohypochondriac; nor does he/she have an inordinate need to verbalize guilt feelings, which is invariably found in true hypochondriasis.

It is not easy to distinguish between hypochondriasis and pseudohypochondriasis in practice, as is evident from the two cases described below. Nevertheless, if one proceeds on the premise that my formulation is accurate, it becomes apparent that a failure to make this distinction may worsen the patient's physiological as well as his/her psychological state.

On his first visit to Dr. R.'s office, Mr. V., who was seventy-five years old, provided a nonstop recitation of his diffuse complaints, including his vision, his hearing, and his urinary system. After a complete physical examination failed to show any physical abnormality, Dr. R.'s suspicions were aroused. When he determined that Mr. V. had none of the other signs or symptoms of a depressive reaction and was able to rule out an organic mental syndrome, he began to give serious consideration to the possibility that Mr. V. might be a hypochondriac. He completed routine laboratory tests on Mr. V. and asked him to return in a week.

When Mr. V. was informed that laboratory test findings were within normal limits, he reacted with great relief. He did not question the accuracy of Dr. R.'s diagnosis, nor did he press for further tests or diagnostic procedures. He did express concern, however, about his behavior. Mr. V. felt that he had "blown up" his physical complaints, "made a mountain out of a molehill," and he insisted that it wasn't like him to behave this way. He went on to confide in Dr. R. that he had always been a "happy-go-lucky" sort, with a fairly optimistic attitude. But his attitude seemed to have changed as he grew older. He had out-lived everyone and everything that had been important to him. Now, instead of focusing on others he focused on himself.

Miss Q.'s behavior was in marked contrast to Mr. V.'s. Miss Q., a sixty-seven-year-old unmarried woman, was seen by Dr. G. only once. He formed a tentative diagnosis of hypochondriasis on the basis of subsequent phone calls and requests for medical information from a variety of sources.

On her first and only visit to Dr. G., Miss Q. presented multiple systemic complaints: She was dizzy, nauseous, had cramps, and she had been experiencing vaginal, rectal, and buccal mucosal burning senstations for 6 months. She also ad-mitted that she had been feeling increasingly depressed and that she lived alone and was estranged from her only living rela-tives. Dr. G.'s first task was to rule out any physiological basis for her complaints, and in fact all findings were within normal lim-its. After informing the patient that he could find nothing wrong with her, Dr. G. suggested that she return for another visit if she didn't feel better within a few weeks.

Dr. G.'s reassurance made little impression on Miss Q. The next day he received a phone call from the emergency room of a neighborhood hospital requesting information on his patient, who had presented with a similar list of complaints, insisted that she felt sick and "limp", and was experiencing palpitations, shortness of breath, chest pain, and syncopal episodes. At this point Miss Q. was hospitalized for a suspected pulmonary em-bolism. In the hospital she was started on anticoagulants. When it became increasingly apparent after further physiological tests that her complaints were primarily psychogenic, Miss Q. was discharged.

In all probability the fact that Miss Q. was told that she had no significant physiological dysfunction, that she was in good condition for her age, did not induce her to give up her "cru-sade." One can speculate that Miss Q. will continue to go from doctor to doctor in a never-ending search for the one physician who can find something seriously wrong with her.

CLINICAL FEATURES

Altman (1975) has succinctly summarized the clinical features of hypochondriasis:

1. Preoccupied with bodily functions
2. Unshakeable belief that physical illness is present out of keeping with physical findings
3. Vague shifting somatic complaints
4. Symptoms exaggerated from physical findings
5. Regressive relationships (limited social life)
6. Dwells on and is proud of suffering
7. History of unsatisfactory medical care
8. Withdrawal from the outside world with the body becoming a substitute for interpersonal relationships

DEVELOPMENT (ONTOGENESIS) OF HYPOCHONDRIASIS

The theoretical development of hypochondriasis in psychodynamic terms can be explained on the basis of a failure in separation-individuation (Mahler, 1968) in two spheres: first, between self and object, and second, between mind and body. Hypochondriasis may result through the mechanism of either regression or fixation and is commonly seen in borderline or extreme narcissistic personality disorders (Kernberg, 1975; Kohut, 1964). It is reminiscent of an undifferentiated preoedipal state where there is not only lack of differentiation between self and other but between the mental self and the body self of the individual (Jacobson, 1964). Richards (1981) has reviewed self theory, conflict theory, and the problem of hypochondriasis: "Self psychologists view hypochondriasis as pathognomonic of the disorders of the self and indicative of self fragmentation and loss of self-cohesion rather than a compromise-impulse-defense constellation." The determinants of individuation include (1) constitution (genetic endowment) and (2) experience (mother-child relationship, trauma, learning).

Experience-nurturing vicissitudes may result in (1) fear of abandonment, (2) a pathological parent-child relationship, and

(3) anger and sustained feelings of guilt. All of these may contribute to foster hypochondriacal thinking. Anger toward the dissapointing object can result in the following:
Aggression → introjection (from fear of object loss) → self → masochism.

Another contribution to the formulation of hypochondriasis—one that is not sufficiently understood—is the patient's need to suffer. Man is traditionally depicted as driven by two overriding desires: the avoidance of pain and the achievement of pleasure. In striking contrast to this popular view of human behavior, the patient who needs to suffer deliberately seeks mental or physical pain (possibly via noncompliance) as a source of unconscious pleasure (Strain, 1978).

The child who, as a consequence of his/her early experiences, is vulnerable to the fear of abandonment may attempt to cope with this fear by deliberately provoking punishment from his parents as a means of gaining their attention and ensuring their interest (Brenner, 1959). In so doing he creates the illusion that he can control his parents—and his fate. When such a relationship continues over time, the child may become convinced that he is most loved when he suffers most. Suffering may then be used as a form of blackmail: He learns that his parents are most responsive when he appears to be unhappy, when he is experiencing physical discomfort or pain, and, most important, when they are made to feel that they are responsible for his plight, that they have failed somehow to fulfill their obligations as parents. Thus, the child not only makes himself suffer, he also makes his parents suffer. This serves an important purpose: When the child makes others suffer, he provokes their wrath and is made to suffer in turn. When the child learns that physical symptoms are the route to controlling, manipulating, and adapting to the environment, these behaviors may become central to coping and to psychological homeostasis.

Second, this behavior may have its roots in the quality of the child's relationship with his parents (Brenner, 1959). If a child is criticized constantly, or if he is treated in a cruel, humiliating, and rejecting manner, in later life he may come to believe that he doesn't deserve any better. He may treat himself badly and expect similar treatment from others or provoke others to treat him in a cruel and rejecting manner.

Third, the need to suffer may derive from sustained feelings of guilt. The young child is under great pressure from his conscience to follow the dictates of his parents and society. When parental prohibitions are excessively harsh or unrealistic, their violation produces overwhelming feelings of guilt, which lay the groundwork for the need to suffer.

Illness and suffering are the means by which the hypochondriac maintains gratifying (albeit ambivalent) relationships. Thus, unlike the malingerer, the hypochondriac actually experiences symptoms, but like the malingerer, his suffering provides important primary gain. Via his suffering the hypochondriac is able to express his unacceptable dependency needs and anger without loss of self-esteem, for the hypochondriac's belief that his illness really does exist protects his self-esteem. Unlike the malingerer, he does not consciously attempt to deceive anyone (Altman, 1975).

By being hypochondriacal the patient gains the physician's attention and interest, which, paradoxically, diminishes the fear of abandonment. If hypochondriacs learned early in life that they are loved most when they suffer most, hypochondriasis may provide them with a royal road toward suffering. At the same time, even while he is experiencing the physical discomfort and pain, he attempts to convince the physician that the responsibility for relieving him is the physician's; that the physician has failed to fulfill his clinical obligation. Furthermore, he provokes the physician via his hypochondriasis with the unconscious hope that the physician will take "revenge." The needs that suffering served in the context of the parent-child relationship are reenacted in the context of the doctor-patient relationship.

Thus, such a patient may refuse to adhere to a treatment regimen of demonstrated efficacy or manifest a "negative therapeutic reaction"; i.e., he may react with hostility to the doctor's reassurance that his chronic illness can be stabilized, discount the possible benefits of any remission, and flee treatment when told there is no evidence of organic pathology. Inevitably, these behaviors give rise to disappointment, disgust, and frustration in the physician, who may then respond, understandably, with anger and rejection: "How can Mr. F. be so damn ungrateful?" "To hell with him; he's going to bitch regardless of what I do." "Let him suffer—that's what he wants anyway."

By refusing to join in the prescribed treatment regimen and to accept that there is no significant physical dysfunction, the patient is able to fulfill his need to suffer. At the same time his hypochondriasis enables him to maintain control over the physician by depriving him of his most precious possession—his therapeutic potency. In short, the physician falls into the patient's "trap" when he/she responds with annoyance and rejection to his behavior, for in so doing he/she fulfills the patient's wishes. The patient is then convinced that it is the doctor who is the difficult one, that he is once again the helpless "victim." Actually, both the patient and his doctor are victims.

In summary, the nature of the patient's object relationship including the relationship with the doctor is (1) ambivalent, (2) masochistic-sadistic, (3) primitive, (4) idealized, (5) egocentric. And the doctor's typical response toward the patient is (1) anger, (2) withdrawal, (3) transfer.

MANAGEMENT

Physicians caring for hypochondriacal patients (Altman, 1975) should follow certain guidelines:

1. Be alert to the possibility of organic illness.
2. Treat the primary psychiatric disorder if present.
3. Never challenge or disparage the symptoms of a hypochondriac.
4. Encourage short, frequent visits not dependent on illness.
5. Maintain continuing interest in the body.
6. Contract for return appointment even if not "sick."
7. Use psychotropic medications conservatively.
8. Be aware that the patient seldom accepts referral to a psychiatrist or follows through with psychiatric treatment.
9. Focus on "caring and adaptation" not on "cure."

First, the expectation that negative physical findings and the attention of a kindly, sympathetic, noncritical doctor will eliminate the patient's hypochondriasis and will enhance his sense of well-being is misguided. Moreover, to hold out the prospect of a diminution of physical suffering will only intensify the patient's anxiety and his aberrant behavior.

Second, the doctor's attempts to introduce the element of reality into the patient's view of his condition will not neccessarily alter his negative and pessimistic orientation. The physician who attempts to change the patient's orientation does not understand that the patient's ability to have a relationship based on suffering enables him to maintain psychological homeostasis.

Third, a therapeutic attitude vis-à-vis such patients would be analogous to that of the parent who must deal reasonably with a sulky, stubborn, provocative child (Brenner, 1959). If the parent is wise and does not allow himself/herself to become over-involved emotionally with the child's behavior, he/she will not be excessively upset or disturbed by such behavior but remain calmly observant and understanding, however seductive the child's efforts to provoke him may be. The physician's relatively limited contact with and emotional investment in the patient who needs to suffer should make this affectively neutral stance at least as feasible for him/her as it is for the parent.

At the same time, although we have stressed the need for the doctor to tolerate such behavior, certain limits should be set in terms of his/her own comfort. The physician is not required to become the patient's victim. He/she is not required to tolerate the patient's tirades in silence, without at least calling it to his attention, nor required to accept calmly the patient's accusations that he/she is incompetent, when the patient's failure to improve is clearly the result of his unconscious psychological needs.

Finally, the maintenance of an ongoing doctor-patient relationship over an extended period of time, a relationship that will not crumble in the face of the patient's repetitive, monotonous expressions of dissatisfaction with his lot in life, that will withstand his refusal to comply with the medical regimen, is the single most important aspect of management. With the hypochondriac, the necessity for the doctor to adapt to his/her patient is probably the rate-limiting factor in management. It is necessary for the doctor to tolerate an ambivalent, dependent, regressed, demanding, hostile, sadomasochistic relationship.

As with the dying patient, the characteristics of the hypochondriac challenge the unconscious fantasies of the physician as the powerful healer, the indestructible self, the destructive force (Spikes & Holland, 1975).

A major determinant of the physician's negative response to the hypochondriacal patient is his fantasy of omnipotence. The physician who believes that he alone has the power to restore the patient to health, or at least to bring about symptom relief, may be frustrated by the patient who deliberately thwarts his efforts to "cure" him. The hypochondriac confronts the physician with the reality that his own body and mind also can be disordered (that he is not indestructible) and that should the doctor give vent to his own anger and despair, he can be a destructive-harmful force to the patient and drive him away.

The hostility the patient's hypochondriasis evokes in the physician is problematic for another reason as well. The physician feels impatient and angry with the patient, but he tries to repress these feelings for he views his impatience and anger as inappropriate and unprofessional. If this conflict cannot be resolved, the doctor may become immobilized or may decide that he no longer wants to be "involved" in the patient's care.

Several approaches to the hypochondriacal patient have been employed in addition to individual treatment by the primary care physician. These include conjoint treatment with a psychiatrist and the primary care physician in the medical setting. Divan and Nesbitt (1978) report the use of regular semiweekly group therapy sessions run by a physician/social worker team for patients who are solely hypochondriacal and who participate on an elective basis. Mally and Ogston (1964) also report the use of groups.

The use of a systems approach for psychosomatic disorders has been described by Minuchin (1974). As is true of the linear approach, the open systems model, as employed by Minuchin, seeks to identify the symptom, the precipitating event, and the factors that maintain the symptom. In contrast to the linear approach, however, Minuchin emphasizes that family interactional patterns, as well as intrapsychic phenomena, may trigger the onset and/or hamper the subsidence of psychophysiological processes, and that illness may disrupt family organization or serve as a homeostatic mechanism that regulates family interactions.

Viewed within the framework of the open systems model, psychological management can be aimed at the patient, the family, the feedback processes inherent in the family's transactional patterns, or all three. Minuchin (1974) sees as the goal of psychological intervention the minimization of the pathogenic force within the family system and of four major pathogenic characteristics in particular: enmeshment, overprotection, rigidity, and lack of conflict resolution. Certainly, family therapy of hypochondriacal patients should be systematically investigated for its effectiveness.

It is important to acknowledge a Buddhist-based treatment for neuroses—Morita psychotherapy—whose goal is not to remove symptoms such as anxieties and phobias but to have them accepted as part of the phenomenological reality of the patient at the moment they are experienced (Reynolds, 1981; Suzuki & Suzuki, 1981).

The ability to learn how to live with symptoms and yet maximize one's life experience has been the basic philosophy of the approach to the hypochondriasis patient expressed in this chapter. Since hypochondriacal patients are as diverse and individual as any patient group, certain subgroups may be more amenable to treatment than are others. As Decker has emphasized, each patient needs to be individually evaluated to ascertain his/her capacity to grow and change; techniques such as skilled empathetic mirroring may promote enhanced adaptation in certain patients (N. Decker, *personal communication,* 1984). Brown and Vaillant (1981) emphasize that hypochondriacal patients are managed best in medical rather than psychiatric settings.

In conclusion, specific measures of success in treating the hypochondriacal patient should include the following:

1. Fewer hospitalizations and less surgery
2. Fewer clinic and emergency room visits
3. Fewer medications and examinations

4. Less emphasis and agitation over somatic symptoms
5. An increase in the patients' reflection on their own be-
    havior and how they contribute to the unpleasant sit-
    uations in which they find themselves

With the juvenile diabetic, if the number of hospitalizations can be reduced during a given year, the pediatrician has
made important progress. The underlying key to the management of the hypochondriac is similar—the need to change from
a model of cure to an adaptational model, one that permits a
disease-compatible life-style.

REFERENCES

Altman, N. (1975). Hypochondriasis. In S. Grossman & J. J. Strain
    (Eds.), *Psychological care of the medically ill: A primer in liaison psychia-
    try.* (pp. 76–93) New York: Appleton-Century-Crofts.
Brenner, C. (1959). The masochistic character: Genesis and treatment.
    Journal of American Psychoanalytic Association, 7, 197.
Brown, H. N., & Vaillant, G. E. (1981). Hypochondriasis. *Archives of
    Internal Medicine, 141,* 723–726.
Busse, E. W. (1982). Hypochondriasis in the elderly. *American Family
    Physician, 2,* 199–202.
Diagnostic and statistical manual of mental disorders, 3d ed. (1980).
    Washington, DC: American Psychiatric Association.
Divan, C., & Nesbitt, J. (1978). Group approach to hypochondriasis.
    American Family Physician, 18, 23.
Ehrlich, R. (1980). *The healthy hypochondriac: Recognizing, understanding
    and living with anxieties about our health.* New York: Saunders Press.
Jacobson, E. (1964). *Self and the object world.* New York: International
    Universities Press.
Kenyon, F. (1964). Hypochondriasis: A clinical study. *British Journal of
    Psychiatry, 110,* 478–488.
Kenyon, F. (1976). Hypochondriacal states. *British Journal of Psychiatry,
    76,* 1–14.
Kernberg, O. (1975). *Borderline conditions and pathological narcissism.* New
    York: Jason Aronson.
Kohut, H. (1964). *The analysis of the self.* New York: International Uni-
    versities Press.

Ladde, G. A. (1966). *Hypochondriacal syndromes.* New York: Elsevier.

Lipsett, D. (1970). Medical and psychological characteristics of "crocks." *Psychiatry Medicine, 1,* 15–27.

Mahler, M. (1968). *On human symbiosis and the viscissitudes of individuation.* New York: International Universities Press.

Mally, M. A., & Ogston, W. D. (1964). Treatment of the untreatables. *International Journal of Psychotherapy, 14,* 369–374.

Mechanic, D. (1973). Social psychologic factors affecting the presentation of bodily complaints. *New England Journal of Medicine, 287,* 1132–1139.

Minuchin, S. (1974). *Families and family therapy.* Cambridge, MA: Harvard University Press.

Munro, A. (1978). Monosymptomatic psychoses manifesting as delusions of parasitoses: Treatment with pimozide G. *Archives of Dermatology, 114,* 940–943.

Palmore, E. (1970). *Normal aging.* Durham, NC: Duke University Press.

Pilowsky, I. (1970). Primary and secondary hypochondriasis. *Acta Psychiatrica Scandinavica, 46,* 273–285.

Reynolds, D. K. (1981). Preface to the effectiveness of in-patient Morita therapy. *Psychiatric Quarterly, 53,* 201.

Richards, A. (1981). Self theory, conflict theory, and the problem of hypochondriasis. *Psychoanalytic Study of the Child, 36,* 319–337.

Spikes, J., & Holland, J. (1975). The physician's response to the dying patient. In J. J. Strain & S. Grossman (Eds.), *Psychological care of the medically ill: A primer in liaison psychiatry.* (pp. 138–150) New York: Appleton-Century-Crofts.

Strain, J. J. (1978). *Psychological interventions in medical practice.* (pp. 91–104, 116–118) New York: Appleton-Century-Crofts.

Suzuki, T., & Suzuki, R. (1981). The effectiveness of in-patient Morita therapy. *Psychiatric Quarterly, 53,* 203.

Turnbull, J. M. (1974). Hypochondriasis. In C. L. Bowden & A. G. Burstein (Eds.), *Psychosocial basis of medical practice.* (pp. 73–80) Baltimore: Williams & Wilkins.

PART II

SURGICAL PROBLEMS

Chapter 7

ACUTE ADJUSTMENT TO TRAUMA

Linda G. Peterson

Trauma patients are confronted with complex emotional and physical problems. These patients have had a recent psychological and physical stress and may be suffering from grief or loss. In many cases these people have preexisting psychological or social problems that predisposed them to becoming trauma patients. In addition they are now also suffering from major physical disabilities, including amputation, major organ system dysfunction, repeated surgeries, and exposure to multiple classes of medication, all of which further affect their psychological and physical functioning. Broader issues in trauma, such as the wide range of posttraumatic stress disorders (acute, chronic, and delayed) and sequelae of large-scale trauma such as that experienced by concentration camp survivors, prisoners of war, Vietnam veterans, or victims of natural disasters will not be discussed in this report. Neither will the question be addressed of who are accident victims in terms of previous psychiatric problems or life stress, although this has been discussed by Rosenbaum (1978) and by other authors. Looking at the epidemiology of trauma victims, the presence of alcoholism, alcohol abuse, and immediate life stress are common and must always be remembered when approaching posttrauma care.

The focus of this discussion will be the individual trauma victim, his/her family, the hospital staff, and the particular psychological problems seen after arrival at the hospital. Also, some general and specific treatment approaches for dealing with these problems will be outlined. Trauma is defined for these purposes as an event characterized by physical injuries severe enough to necessitate at least a week of hospitalization. (I will exclude trauma associated with intentional acts of self or others.) Injuries may include multiple fractures, amputations, burns, damaged internal organs, or head injury. As a part of the trauma-causing event, the individual may have seen friends, co-workers, or family members injured or even killed. As has been described in bereavement responses (Lindemann, 1944), responses to death and dying (Kubler-Ross, 1975), and posttraumatic stress responses (Horowitz, 1973, 1974), patients responding to trauma typically pass through various phases of adjustment. These phases will be modified by the event, the other losses the patients have suffered, previous psychiatric problems or personality traits, family and other social support, and last but not least, the severity of injury and the course of recovery. In outline, these phases include (1) confusion, (2) shock, (3) denial, (4) depression and anger, and (5) recovery.

PERIOD OF CONFUSION

These phases are not the same as those reported for posttraumatic stress disorders, because for most hospitalized patients there is a period before they are able to comprehend what has happened to them. This is the period I have called the period of confusion. At this time the patient may have had multiple surgeries, may be on a number of medications for pain, and for other reasons may be unable to comprehend cognitively and respond emotionally to the sequelae of his trauma. He also may have metabolic derangements secondary to his injuries, which impair his cognitive functioning and affective state. The result is a period in which the patient perceives pieces of the event that has occurred and its impact. He may or may not realize the full significance of his injuries. He may or may not be aware of what happened during the accident. In fact, large memory gaps surrounding the time of the event may be present, particularly if the patient had any head trauma. During this stage of partial comprehension, rarely does the patient demonstrate significant psychological responses to the trauma.

In this phase, psychiatric help may be needed to manage delirium or psychotic symptoms of behavior related to delirious states. These usually require careful evaluation of metabolic factors, medication, the presence of head trauma, the presence of infection, and factors that might predispose the patient to a brief reactive psychosis. Sometimes symptomatic treatment with low-dose antipsychotic agents is warranted for these conditions as well as correction of the etiologic medical problems. Three problems that need particular attention during this period are psychiatric symptoms secondary to (1) multiple anticholinergic medications given for pain, for sleep, and for gastrointestinal problems, (2) alcohol withdrawal, and (3) head trauma, such as labile mood, agitation, hallucinations, and delusions. The following case is a good example of the conjunction of a number of these problems.

Case No. 1

Mr. M. was a forty-year-old married white male engineer with a major corporation who was involved in a motor vehicle accident. He sustained multiple fractures and possible frontal lobe contusion. The patient lost consciousness for an unknown period of time, probably less than 24 h and since then had been agitated and confused. There was a drinking history of two to three bourbon-and-waters a night but no past sequelae of alcohol abuse. He was placed immediately on Librium®, 75 mg, q.i.d.; Dilantin®, 100 mg, t.i.d.; Tylenol®, #3, 1 to 2 tablets every 4 h; and thiamine.

On interview the patient was intermittently somnolent and agitated. He could follow simple commands but could not give more than one-word answers to questions; he would give his own name and his wife's but was otherwise totally disoriented. He could not recall three objects even at 1 min and had no memory for recent events. He could not name common objects. He had no hallucinations or delusions. He was felt to have an organic brain syndrome with possible aphasia.

Three etiologies were suggessted: (1) delirium tremens, (2) head trauma, (3) paradoxical reaction to Librium—or some combination of the foregoing. Since the patient had shown no improvement on Librium, it was discontinued, and the patient was placed on Haldol®, 5 mg every 2 h as needed. This decreased agitation somewhat, and after a month Mr. M.'s behavior was moderately improved. He was oriented times three but still had gross memory and judgment impairment and was just learning to comprehend the sequelae of his injury. This case is typical of the early posttraumatic period.

Once the phase of confusion has passed, emotional outcry may ensue when the full realization of what has happened hits the patient for the first time. Symptoms experienced may include depression, anger, anxiety, numbness, and nightmares. However, these injured patients, unlike those who are physically unharmed after a major traumatic event, may never experience full emotional outcry as one coherent episode but may have smaller, more disjunctive states of dysphoria, distress, irritability or uncontrolled crying. When this first appears, the staff often sees this as evidence of psychiatric difficulty, since up until now the patient has been quiet and cooperative and has not been a management problem. Consultation at this time most often necessitates assessment of the appropriateness of the patient's outbursts, along with attention to the staff's distress over the episodes. Reassurance of both staff and patient is helpful, as is reconstructing the event and its impact on the patient with the patient himself.

SHOCK AND NUMBNESS

Of more concern are those patients who experience no obvious outcry at the time that the full impact of their injury and losses are first made known to them. These patients may pass directly into the next phase of shock and numbness. They may express distress over their losses and yet have difficulty experiencing the feelings associated with them. Many of these people ask to see a psychiatrist because of their feeling that their lack of emotion is inhuman or unnatural.

Case No. 2

Mrs. B. was a thirty-year-old married white female nurse who was in a serious motorcycle accident 3 weeks prior to consultation. Her husband was killed in the same accident. Mrs. B. suffered head trauma and had no memory of the accident. She *knew* that her husband was dead and that he was still *unburied* in a funeral home in another town. She had deliberately avoided talking about her husband because she had been afraid that she would "lose my mind." The day prior to consultation she decided that she was making herself worse by trying to avoid grieving, so she asked to see a psychiatrist. She stated she was ready to start talking about her husband's death and let herself grieve. Despite saying this, Mrs. B. would only intermittently be willing to talk about her husband. Often she would say talking about him made her headaches worse and refuse to go on. On several occasions she spent hours crying, which she later recognized as related to grief for her husband and for her own physical losses. At other times she had fights with the nurses over trivial matters. She realized later that her losses made her resent the healthy nurses who took care of her. Even after discharge her ability to deal with grieving was sporadic until 3 months post-injury.

In instances like this one patients who remain for a prolonged period of time in this state of numbness often have feelings that they were personally responsible for the death or disability of others involved in the accident, whether this is realistic or not. Mrs. B., for example, felt that she was responsible for her husband's death—she had had to ask him to take her to visit a patient because her car was not running. During this period problems with dreams of the accident or other distressing feelings about the event are common. At times, if sleep disturbance and posttraumatic dreaming is excessive, low-dose tricyclic antidepressant medication may allow better verbalization of grief. It did for Mrs. B. After a matter of weeks most patients pass through this phase into one of oscillating depression and anger.

DEPRESSION AND ANGER

Some patients will have mostly angry responses, depending on the traumatic event, their previous personality traits, and their responses to stress in the past. In fact, one study of trauma patients found significantly more hostility among these patients than among other groups of hospitalized patients (Kane, 1977). Other patients may appear primarily depressed and sad. Key factors in this stage are the duration of hospitalization, the degree of disability, the other losses suffered during the traumatic event, and the amount of emotional support available from staff, family, and friends. Several patients with whom we have been asked to consult have been particularly angry because they were the victims of the carelessness of a drunk driver or because they have felt no control over their injury. Depression has been most common among patients who have been hospitalized a long time with ambiguous prognoses that continuously were being revised. Often they have had repeated surgeries over a period of months to years and were unclear about whether they ever would recover fully.

Case No. 3

Mr. L. was a twenty-seven-year-old married white male, whose wife was killed in the accident in which his own leg was crushed. With multiple grafts, use of a Hoffman device, and several other surgeries, an attempt was made to save his leg, resulting in more than six long hospitalizations in the subsequent year. Intitially, Mr. L. asked to see a psychiatrist to talk about his anger over his wife's death and the careless driver responsible. He also was concerned about his leg and described some past difficulty with drug use in the service. As the question of the viability of his leg became less and less clear and he was repeatedly hospitalized and on bed rest, he began to be abusive to the staff, often threatening to leave against medical advice, demanding drugs, and stating that he didn't care if he was addicted. After an amputation 1 year later he returned to work and school and has had no further emotional problems.

Other patients who seem to have particular difficulties are those with little social support because they are some distance from their family or for other reasons do not have family or friends available to assist them in the recovery process. During both the shock-and-numbness phase and the depression-and-anger phase it is helpful to review and reconstruct the accident, the feelings around it, the thoughts, the remembrances of the early parts of the hospitalization, and what has been told to them by other people involved. It allows adequate expression of emotions and connecting of those feelings and thoughts, which by now have become dissociated. Again, in those patients who seem to have more severe problems with depression, treatment with antidepressents and brief psychotherapy can be helpful.

PERIOD OF RECOVERY

Finally, in the recovery period many patients, once they have a fixed date for leaving the hospital, seem to go through a period of extreme psychological rejuvenation. For those with minimal residual deficits this may persist and be the prelude to return to normal psychological adjustment. For others there is a posthospital letdown when they arrive home and find that their limitations are still there and that the losses they had experienced and begun to deal with in the hospital are now more intensively experienced. Residual problems in these patients become more typical of those seen in posttraumatic stress disorders, chronic and delayed types. For many patients blocked or incomplete grief reactions are present, because they were in the hospital at the time when loved ones died and were buried. The grieving that went on communally with other family and relatives was therefore unavailable to the patient.

THERAPEUTIC INTERVENTIONS

Having discussed the various phases of response to trauma in these patients, it is important to look at therapeutic modalities that may be needed. These include psychopharmacologic agents, psychotherapeutic intervention, and social or environmental intervention. Starting with the psychopharmacologic agents, those patients who have marked emotional lability, nightmares, and disturbances in mood during the acute phases of response to grief respond to antidepressant medication, particularly imipramine in doses of 25 mg or 50 mg at night. It often decreases nightmares and mood lability, allowing a more constructive approach to grief (Marshall, 1975). Typically, these agents need only be continued for 2 or 3 weeks during the acute phase, whereas patients with posttraumatic stress disorders seem to require longterm use of the antidepressants. For posttraumatic nightmares, imipramine has proved efficacious, as have monoamine oxidase (MAO) inhibitors. However, because of the dietary restrictions required when using MAO inhibitors they are second choices. Although patients recovering from trauma often have a significant number of medical problems, there have rarely been occasions in which antidepressants at this dosage level have caused any difficulty, either with hypotension or with other anticholinergic or cardiac side effects. If they cannot be used in an oral form, then amitriptyline, 25 mg or 50 mg, intramuscularly, can be used. Patients with psychotic reactions or delirium who require treatment of their agitation, hallucinations, and delusions may be placed on haloperidol in doses of 1 mg if they are mildly agitated (hourly until they are sedated) or 5 mg if they are more severely agitated. This can be given orally or intramuscularly, or it can be administered intravenously to patients with poor cardiac output who may not absorb the drug intramuscularly and cannot take it orally. When used intravenously, 1 to 2 mg every 30 to 60 min until sedation is achieved is usually an adequate dose. Another drug that can be used in this context is droperidol (Ayd, 1980), usually in a 10-mg dose, either intramuscularly or intravenously. The major problems with droperidol may be mild transient hypotension and reflex tachycardia. These do not appear to be problems with haloperidol (Dudley, Rowlett, & Loebel, 1979), though laryngospasms have been reported. Use of either of these agents acutely can be followed by a regimen of once-a-day therapy, using a ratio of two-thirds of the 24-h dose that was required to maintain the patient in a calm state. During this period the etiology for the psychotic symptoms should be assessed carefully. Electrolyte imbalances, infection, or intracranial processes such as unrecognized subdural hematoma or bleed, which might be the causal factors of the delirium, are particularly frequent and should be corrected immediately.

We have used these same agents in patients with closed head trauma who develop agitation and uncontrollable behavior, although some caution may be in order because of a recent report of decreased relearning of skills in mice given haloperidol after brain damage (Feeney, Gonzalez, & Law, 1982).

Psychotherapeutic interventions usually have been of two types: intervention to deal with grief and intervention to deal with posttraumatic stress responses and adjustment to disability.

The intervention for grief usually has included a review of the relationship and history of the patient and the dead person, together with an attempt to talk about those things the patient wishes he/she had been able to say to the dead person. Frequently, patients also wish to discuss ways in which they may formalize their grieving, such as holding memorial services after they leave the hospital or creating some type of memorial to the deceased person and in this way participate more actively in the grieving. This is often an effective substitute for the grieving that family and friends were able to do through the funeral and burial, which the hospitalized patient had missed. Often such patients will require further therapy once they leave the hospital, because returning home and dealing with the loss at home again awakens very strong feelings that the rest of the family is no longer experiencing.

For those patients who are experiencing posttraumatic stress syndrome and difficulty adjusting to complications of their injuries, the psychotherapeutic approach begins by reviewing their social and vocational situation prior to injury and their life's accomplishments and goals, and then reviewing the memory of the accident, hospitalization, and the affects they have experienced since in relation to these events. Finally, looking at constructive ways in which they may return to vocational and social usefulness can be effective. This can be accomplished usually in six to eight sessions. For those patients with preexisting psychiatric problems and those with depression or alcoholism, more in-depth therapy and treatment of these problems may be required. However, many patients, once they understand their personality style, can connect their feelings and thoughts and fit the traumatic event into their world view with brief therapeutic intervention. This technique has been outlined clearly by Horowitz (1973, 1974) and can be utilized effectively in this group of patients.

CONCLUSIONS

The major conclusion in dealing with patients who are trauma victims is that careful attention must be paid to (1) the phase they are in post trauma, (2) the presence of grief reactions along with response to injury, (3) the presence of pre-existing psychiatric problems, particularly alcoholism or depression, (4) the degree of responsibility the patients feel for the traumatic event, (5) the complications that will ensue from the event, and finally, (6) the potential recovery period and the amount of support available from family and friends throughout the recovery period.

The approaches outlined for dealing with posttraumatic stress disorders based on personality style and for intervention with patients experiencing acute grief are important tools in working with trauma patients. The use of antidepressants, particularly in those patients who seem to have excessive depression symptoms and/or blocked grief that is unresponsive to psychotherapeutic intervention, is often helpful. The use of low-dose antipsychotic medications during periods of delirium, or if brief reactive psychoses appear, also may facilitate recovery.

Trauma patients are some of the most challenging to work with and some of the most rewarding. The importance of appropriate psychological intervention cannot be overstated, as numerous studies have demonstrated that psychosocial factors play a central role in rehabilitation.

REFERENCES

Ayd, F. J. (1980). Parenteral (IM/IV) droperidol for acutely disturbed behavior in psychotic and non-psychotic individuals. *International Drug Therapy Newsletter, 15,* 3.

Dudley, D. L., Rowlett, D. B., & Loebel, P. J. (1979). Emergency use of intravenous haloperidol. *General Hospital Psychiatry, 1,* 240–246.

Feeney, D. M., Gonzalez, A., & Law, W. A. (1982). Amphetamine, haloperidol, and experience interact to affect rate of recovery after motor cortex injury. *Science, 217,* 855–857.

Horowitz, M. J. (1973). Phase oriented treatment of stress response syndromes. *American Journal of Psychotherapy, 27,* 506–515.

Horowitz, M. J. (1974). Stress response syndromes. *Archives of General Psychiatry, 31,* 718–781.

Kane, M. (1977). *Hostility reactions in trauma patients.* Unpublished master's thesis, Texas Women's University, Denton, TX.

Kubler-Ross, E. (1975). *Death: The final stage of growth.* Englewood Cliffs, NJ: Prentice Hall.

Lindemann, E. (1944). Symptomatology and management of acute grief. *American Journal of Psychiatry, 101,* 141–148.

Marshall, J. R. (1975). The treatment of night terrors associated with the posttraumatic syndrome. *American Journal of Psychiatry, 132,* 3.

Rosenbaum, J. F. (1978). The accident victim. In T. P. Hackett & N. H. Cassem (Eds.), *Massachusetts General Hospital handbook of general hospital psychiatry.* (pp. 380–391) St. Louis: C. V. Mosby.

Chapter 8

PSYCHOLOGICAL ASPECTS OF CORONARY BYPASS SURGERY

Richard S. Blacher

It is hard to imagine a medical procedure more fraught with anxiety for the patient than surgery on the heart. As surgical techniques have improved, mortality rates have plummeted, and coronary bypass operations have become more and more an everyday occurrence at many medical centers. More than 100,000 are performed in the country each year. Yet for the patient the anxiety such an operation evokes has no connection with the safety of the procedure. Because the heart occupies a unique position in the psychic life of man, surgery on this organ becomes an experience for the patient that is qualitatively different from any other surgery. It is a procedure that, although quite often elective, nevertheless carries with it as background the threat of death. The heart, after all, is the central organ of the body and historically the seat of the emotions. It is the only organ that functions in a dramatic on-off mode; if it beats one lives, and if it stops one dies.

This definition of life as equated with the cessation of heartbeat is the prevalent one in our society despite the more scientific resort to EEG findings. The heart, not the brain, is seen as the indicator of life and death. Thus, the patient undergoing cardiac surgery has a different emotional task from that of the patient dealing with surgery on any other organ. Generally, in surgery one fears that one will die while anesthetized; that is, one's heart will stop. The informed cardiac patient faces another problem: he/she must accept the fact that during the operation his/her heart will be stopped and then restarted. In other words, by the usual societal standards he/she will be dead and then brought back to life. This is a heavy psychic burden indeed for the patient. Most patients deal with the anticipation of surgery by massive denial. This does not always succeed. For example, a sophisticated surgeon described how he had spent his preoperative night lying awake contemplating his own heart surgery. "I know very well how the pump operates, but I could not get out of my mind the fact that although the machine would keep all of my vital functions going, with my heart stopped I would be really dead."

This concept of life depending on the heartbeat is seen in another context as well, when a cardiac arrest is reported in the newspaper. It is not uncommon for the headline to state that the patient had died and was brought back to life by a physician.

Because of our cardiocentric view of life, there is a universal statistic that patients consider concerning the danger of surgery, namely, 50 percent. This 50-50 chance they give themselves seems to reflect both the great danger they anticipate in surgery and their view of how the heart functions: it either beats or it doesn't. Interestingly, when one asks patients how they view the danger before surgery, one will hear them parroting the surgeon's figures. When the ordeal is over, however, the patient often expresses the true fear—the 50-50 percentage. How such a view of danger is dealt with in specific situations I will talk about later.

In our institution all patients undergoing coronary bypass are seen by psychiatrists before and after surgery. Although most patients successfully deny dangers and come to surgery calmly (the evening before surgery most patients look as if they were anticipating a golf game the next day), a number of patients develop a great deal of anxiety; and ideally, this anxiety should be reduced in order to have the patient come to surgery in a relaxed state. If this can be brought about, the patient is not only comfortable but will require less anesthetic agent. Most patients are able to deny successfully, and this denial should not be interfered with. Therefore, preoperative exploration is generally best kept to a minimum except in the face of a good deal of anxiety. A staff attitude of quiet efficiency tends to support the patient's denial.

PREOPERATIVE PERIOD

For discussion I have divided the patient's hospitalization into three parts: preoperative, intraoperative, and postoperative. The preoperative period begins when the patient is notified that he/she will be scheduled for surgery. Depending on the patient's personality and the time he/she must wait for the operation, this period may be one of great tension. Unlike an eminent cardiac surgeon (*Medical World News,* 1976) who was able to dictate immediate surgery for himself when his catheterization showed that this was necessary, most patients must wait a number of weeks. For a typical type A person this may be no easy matter. However, when immediate surgery is offered, the time may be too short for the patient to make an easy emotional adaptation to the procedure. Many patients are able to push awareness of the upcoming surgery out of their conscious awareness. Interestingly, as the time for surgery approaches, in the last few days there is a change—sometimes gradual and sometimes dramatic—in the lowering of anxiety as the patient's denial comes into play. If the anxiety level does not fall, I believe it is important that a psychiatric intervention be made for the purpose of alleviation. In my experience the causes of preoperative anxiety are rather limited. Only a few patients suffer from anxiety concerning the actual risk, and some patients may have a history of knowing a friend or family member who died shortly after surgery. However, I believe the most common cause of severe anxiety before cardiac surgery centers around a specific fantasy. It usually occurs in someone raised in a religion in which the concept of an afterlife is strongly geographical—that is, where heaven is anticipated to be a very specific place.

One such patient was a forty-six-year-old chemist who came for consultation because of her disabling ambivalence over a suggested coronary bypass. Her severe angina pectoris made active life impossible, yet for reasons she could not understand she was sure she would die during the surgery she so eagerly desired. Raised in a religious family, she had given up her religion during her middle teens over her father's objections. Her mother had died of heart disease when she was ten, and she spoke warmly of their close relationship. As an only child she was doted on by both parents, but it was her mother who was the special person in her life. She talked of her knowledge of the surgical procedure and kept returning to the starting and stopping of her heart: "When the heart stops, it is dead; not you but your heart." When in the second hour she began to reminisce about her wonderful early experiences with her mother, I suggested that the fear of surgery was due to her fantasy that when her heart was stopped her soul would leave her body, go to heaven, and join her dead mother. Then when the surgeon restarted her heart, she would be in conflict between staying in heaven with her mother or returning to life. To this rather wild-sounding interpretation she responded with an eager nod and stated, "You hit it on the head." She was relieved that it was something that someone could talk about, and after this discussion she could accept the operation calmly.

Another patient, a sixty-year-old housewife, was quite anxious preoperatively. She spontaneously reported a dream of the night before in which her older sister, a rather dependent spinster, had appeared to her in an uncharacteristically angry way and said to her, "I can't tell you how hurt I am that you are letting me down this way." She then described, at my prompting, her concept of the operation and noted herself that, "when the heart is stopped, it is like being dead." When I suggested to her that she was worried that at that point she would visit her sister in heaven, she remarked, "But I plan to come back to my husband!" The anticipation that her sister would be angry at her for leaving her and returning to life was the source of her anxiety. When she decided that her sister could wait for her to join her permanently, the anxiety subsided and the patient was able to face her surgery calmly.

In the cases cited above, what I did was merely put into words a fantasy that was already conscious or close to consciousness in the patient. My spelling it out gave the patient permission to discuss what she felt to be something that could not be discussed without embarrassment. The relief on being able to talk about these thoughts was quite evident.

INTRAOPERATIVE PERIOD

Because the use of succinylcholine may make the level of anesthesia difficult to determine, an occasional patient has emerged from the anesthetic state during or at the end of his/her surgery and unfortunately has been awake while paralyzed. This was drawn to our attention years ago, in the early days of cardiac surgery, when we began to note a traumatic neurotic syndrome (Meyer & Blacher, 1961; Blacher, 1975) in certain patients who would wake from sleep complaining of anxiety and irritability, preoccupation with death, and repetitive nightmares that made a return to sleep impossible. These patients would be brought to our attention by the night nurses, who noted the patients wandering around the corridors mumbling about not being sure whether they were dead or alive. The nightmares often would be poorly disguised versions of the operative situation. For example, "I was strapped on the kitchen table and the Mafia was sticking wires into me."

Such a case was a fifty-five-year-old man who was extremely anxious and irritable following coronary bypass done under anesthesia with thiopental, nitrous oxide, and a mixture of droperidol and fentanyl along with curare and succinylcholine. He had repeated dreams of being tied down and unable to move. The explanation that he had been awake during surgery and paralyzed was sufficient to cure the symptoms.

These patients are often quite reluctant to talk to the medical staff lest they be thought insane. This worry about insanity is enhanced by the sense of loss of reality when such a patient wakes in the middle of the night and isn't sure whether he/she is dead or alive.

What seems important in these cases is the awful state of helplessness, when clearly, in the mind of the patient, something must have gone terribly wrong or else he/she would not be awake. The repeated dream can be seen as an attempt to master during sleep what was experienced as overwhelming during the state of being awake (Freud, 1955). We know that patients can tolerate paralysis when awake, from operative subjects whose anesthesia is mainly morphine. They are able to be paralyzed and suffer no apparent psychic difficulty. During surgery the anesthesiologist talks continually to them. Of course we also do not see dramatic reactions to operations done with spinal anesthesia. Because the element of unreality in such a situation is so strong, when the patients are informed that they indeed must have been awake during some part of the procedure, the result is a complete cure of the symptoms.

POSTOPERATIVE PERIOD

Following surgery the patient must face the ordeal of treatment in an intensive care unit (ICU). The atmosphere of such a unit has been described by many writers. Essentially immobilized and surrounded by an array of complicated machinery, the patient has drains and tubes in every orifice and in numerous man-made orifices as well. He/she is completely dependent for comfort and even life itself on his medical attendants. There is massive sensory overstimulation. Those who have described a sensory deprivation for the patient really may be describing the reactions to the monotonous sounds that are experienced by the staff. The patient is in a different position. First, he/she quite naturally has a massive psychological regression from being in such a tenuous and dependent state. Because of this narcissistic position, all stimuli that he/she is aware of in the unit are experienced as pertaining to him/her. In addition, the immobilization itself creates a situation of increasing anxiety with no opportunity to dissipate such tensions by means of physical activity. In the immediate postoperative period the clouded sensorium from the analgesics and from the transient organic mental state that results from cardiopulmonary bypass may act as a calming influence. The main comfort, however, comes from a sensitive nursing staff.

In many ways the ICU might be thought of as the new standard of ambivalence. If one's life is in danger, one wants to be in the safest place; but being in the ICU indicates that one's life is in danger, so one is eager to be out. Occasionally, leaving the unit fairly early can result in an increased amount of anxiety. Stepdown units are most useful in gradually decompressing the patient.

A common hazard of surgical ICUs is a state of paranoia that frequently is not expressed openly but is evident in the furtive, suspicious glances of many patients. The dynamics of this condition are involved with the fact that the treatments that are often the most important for the patient's well-being following cardiac surgery are also often painful or uncomfortable. These include encouraging the patient to take deep breaths against a sternal incision and to move around rather than lie still and guard one's wound, and tracheal suction (perhaps the most uncomfortable treatment of all). These are things that the patient realizes are necessary for him to survive. Nevertheless, at this point he would rather lie still and be left alone. He thus finds himself increasingly angry at his attendants and in what he thinks is a dangerous dilemma. He cannot allow himself to be angry, since he recognizes the necessity for treatment and his dependence on the nurses for life. He also fears that if he is angry, the staff will be angry in return and perhaps allow him to die. In this state he projects his rage and thinks that the nurses want to kill him—a paranoid reaction. This mechanism also makes understandable the nurses' painful ministrations. We do not see this reaction in *our* ICUs very often, and I believe that this is due to the fact that our nurses and I encourage the patients to resent their treatment: "You are not going to like what I'm going to do, but I'm going to do it because it is necessary." This gives the patient permission to be angry and makes unnecessary the need to project. The motto we use is "You don't have to like this; you just have to take it." In case paranoia does develop, we discuss with the patient our understanding of his resentment at what is happening to him, and this may tend to mitigate the condition.

The rate of massive psychic upheaval in ICUs decreased considerably from the early days of cardiac surgery. I believe this has less to do with improved surgical technics and more to do with an expectation of the medical staff concerning the dangers involved in the operation. In the early days of surgery, patients were treated as if they were delicate pieces of porcelain, and the nursing staff was quite anxious in its concern that the patient might die. As surgical technics have improved and mortality rates have dropped, the staff now is quite casual in its expectation that the patient will live. This calm assurance is transmitted to the patient.

I have never been convinced that there is such an entity as an "ICU psychosis." My first work with such patients occurred in a large ICU that housed patients with myocardial infarctions, chest surgery, and cardiac surgery. We rarely saw psychosis in coronary and lung patients, whereas almost all of our cardiac surgery patients when carefully examined exhibited large degrees of psychological difficulty (Blacher, 1972). Thus, all of the patients shared a common ICU, but the psychic upheaval was associated only with the medical condition.

A common problem for patients who have been on cardiopulmonary bypass is the almost universal mental difficulty they exhibit for a varying period of time after the surgery. On simple mental status testing almost every patient shows a significant deficit for the first week or so after surgery in comparison to the preoperative examination. This is not surprising in light of the current status of the bypass apparatus and the brain microembolization resulting from the filtration system (Editorial, *Lancet,* 1982). About 25 to 30 percent of all coronary surgery patients will show some mental difficulty *beforehand* when tested, suggesting that the vascular disease is not limited to the coronary vessels but extends to the brain and other organs as well. Such patients have been shown to have greater difficulty after surgery and a poorer medical prognosis (Rabiner & Wilner, 1980).

It is important postoperatively to identify this organic state for patients so that they may be reassured that the impaired mental functioning is only temporary and that they may expect a return to status quo ante within a short time. Since patients do not know this, they worry that the condition is permanent, and we have seen patients with anxiety and depression centering around this concern.

The most common psychic difficulty after coronary surgery is postoperative depression (Blacher, 1978; Blacher & Cleveland, 1980). Since depressed patients tend to eat poorly, move around too little, and take too much analgesic medication when their symptoms take the form of pain, this psychic state is not a benign condition. It may be potentially lethal and certainly may interfere with the patient's recovery. The frequency of the depression ranges in our experience from 6 to 15 percent. This is purely dependent on the history of the patient, since in most cases the cause of the depression is a sense of guilt related to survival. Typically, the patients become depressed about 3 days after surgery, when many of the major tubes and support systems are removed, and they realize that they will live. On questioning, such patients reveal that they had not expected to survive the surgery. Almost invariably, depressed patients give a history of having had someone in their family who died of heart disease at an age younger than they are themselves. Before coronary surgery was done, a valvulotomy patient who became depressed would have a history of someone in his family having died of a relatively unimportant medical condition compared to his own. There would be a history of siblings who died after appendectomy or following the removal of a benign tumor, for example. With the advent of coronary surgery we began to see patients whose families had a history of coronary disease, and some of our patients were the sole survivors after everyone else had died of the condition.

The dynamics of this depression are involved with survival guilt. In our society death is looked on in a "quantitative" way. This view holds that nature demands a certain number of deaths, and thus if one person dies, another can be spared. This was seen, for example, in war neuroses developing in soldiers whose comrades had been killed in a foxhole. The surviving soldier would become depressed, and an exploration would reveal the theme of "If someone had to die, I'm glad it wasn't I." This was followed by guilt because it was tantamount to feeling, "I'm glad *he* died." After cardiac surgery such patients begin to feel that the death of the other family members has somehow saved *them*.

A fifty-year-old salesman was profoundly depressed after surgery and began spontaneously to talk to the psychiatrist about his dying of pneumonia although he was asymptomatic. He quickly revealed the origin of his fear when he talked of his family. His father had died in a flu epidemic when the patient was two years old, and his mother had died of pneumonia when he was seven, leaving the patient and three other sons. They were all raised by various relatives. About 15 years before, his youngest brother had died of a heart attack. The oldest brother suffered a similar fate 8 years later. Only 1 month before this surgery his remaining brother had died of cancer. Following these deaths, the patient had been sad but not depressed. When surgery was recommended for disabling angina pectoris, he eagerly agreed, not revealing to the doctors that he never thought he would live through the operation. When I suggested that his depression now was paradoxical, since he *had* in fact lived, he talked about not wanting to live at all. At the same time he felt that if he died he would be deserting his children and his wife (as he himself had been deserted). He discussed his sense of guilt over surviving everyone else in the family. When I pointed out to him that it would be very hard to feel like celebrating his success in surviving the operation when others close to him had died, he nodded vigorously. A half-hour later he was noted to be markedly improved, and by the next day his depression had completely gone.

A sixty-year-old man became deeply depressed following his surgery. He had never had any depressive difficulties before. He related that he had not expected to live through surgery, and then he began, with great sadness, to talk of the death of his father from a heart attack when the father was fifty-five. Although outwardly cordial, the relationship of son and father was marked by the son's frustration at the father's dominating him in the business they mutually operated. When it was pointed out to the patient that his depression was paradoxical since he had not expected to live through surgery, he responded plaintively, "They didn't have these operations twenty-five years ago, did they?" He seemed relieved to hear that this was true, and he accepted my statement that it was natural to compare his good fortune with the unfortunate outcome suffered by his father. Within an hour his mood had brightened and he was completely free of symptoms in a few days.

Many patients are completely asymptomatic within minutes of their interviews. These depressions are very amenable to treatment by discussion and do not need, in my experience, antidepressant medication. If untreated, some patients may spontaneously recover from the gross symptoms of depression but maintain a low-level depressive affect.

CORONARY VERSUS VALVE SURGERY

The first cardiotomy psychoses were described in relation to mitral commisurotomy, which at first carried a high rate of psychosis (Fox, Rizzo, & Gifford, 1954). When open heart procedures were done, some observers felt that the rate of psychological difficulties was determined by a number of organic factors, including the length of bypass time (Kornfeld, Zimberg, & Malm, 1965). However, it was observed by many that coronary patients seem to have an easier time psychologically, despite the fact that their pump time was longer by 50 percent than that of patients having a single valve replacement. Although all cardiac surgery is often referred to as "open heart surgery," patients make it clear that they are relieved not to have their hearts opened. We are currently studying both the psychological and the physiological effect of varying the way in which a coronary procedure is described to the patient. Our hypothesis is that a truthful explanation, presented in a calming way preoperatively, may make the postoperative course smoother. It is often little appreciated how difficult it is for the patient to conceptualize the opening of his own heart (Blacher, 1971). Since coronary surgery does not involve such a measure, it may be useful for the patient to have this spelled out in greater detail than is done at many centers.

Perhaps the greatest psychological danger to our coronary bypass patients is our becoming inured to the magnitude of these procedures from the patient's point of view. As these operations become more and more commonplace, we may tend to treat them as if they were minor surgery. Although this may have a calming effect, as I have noted before, if carried too far it may separate us from an awareness of the plight of the person undergoing surgery. This would be detrimental both to the patient and to our function as healers of the sick.

Conclusions

In summary, coronary bypass surgery is now a common procedure. All surgery on the heart provokes intense anxiety because of the unique psychological meaning attached to the heart. Preoperative anxiety is usually contained effectively by denial, but a few patients have the fantasy of dying and temporarily rejoining a dead relative. When this fantasy is elicited and discussed, the anxiety is greatly relieved. Anxiety over the events of the operative period is often related to the patient having been partially conscious during surgery; such patients are concerned that they must be insane because they believe they could not actually have heard what they recall. This anxiety is quickly resolved by the reassurance that they could indeed have been partly aware of what happened. Anxiety in the postoperative period is common in ICUs and is partly related to a transient clouded sensorium. Many patients in this situation recognize their impaired mental state and fear that it is permanent. Reassurance that it will be temporary is effective in relieving the anxiety. Much anxiety in intensive care is related to the intrinsic and intense ambivalence of the situation: being there means one's life is in danger, so one needs to be in a safe place; at the same time one wants to be out of intensive care because being there means one is in danger. The attitude of the nursing and medical staff regarding survival is therefore crucial; if their behavior communicates confidence that the patient will live, such anxiety is greatly relieved.

Paranoid reactions are also common in ICUs. This is related to the need for activity by the patient when he feels like lying still and to the intense activity around him and with him when he feels like being alone. Recognizing the patient's right to be angry and to express it is effective in reducing the paranoia. The most common postoperative psychic problem is depression. This is often related to guilt at having survived when important others have died. Clarifying this often results in dramatic and rapid improvement. Careful and detailed explanation of the actual surgical procedure preoperatively may reduce psychic distress before and after surgery. Finally, we must guard against the risk that we physicians will become inured to the magnitude of heart surgery for the patient because for us it is now so common and because it usually has a good outcome.

REFERENCES

Blacher, R. S. (1971). Open-heart surgery: The patient's point of view. *The Mount Sinai Journal of Medicine, 38,* 74–78.

Blacher, R. S. (1975). On awakening paralyzed during surgery. *Journal of the American Medical Association, 234,* 67–68.

Blacher, R. S. (1978). Paradoxical depression after heart surgery: A form of survivor syndrome. *The Psychoanalytic Quarterly, 47,* 267–283.

Blacher, R. S., & Cleveland, R. J. (1980). Paradoxical depression after open-heart surgery. In H. Speidel & G. Rodewald (Eds.), *Psychic and neurological dysfunctions after open-heart surgery.* (pp. 141–143) New York: Thieme Stratton.

Brain damage after open-heart surgery. (1982). [Editorial]. *Lancet, 1,* 1161–1163.

Fox, H. M., Rizzo, N. D., & Gifford, S. (1954). Psychological observations of patients undergoing mitral surgery: A study of stress. *Psychosomatic Medicine, 16,* 186.

Freud, S. (1955). *Beyond the pleasure principle.* Standard Edition (p. 32). London: Hogarth Press.

A heart surgeon tells of his own coronary bypass. *Medical World News.* October, 1976 (p. 52).

Kornfeld, D. S., Zimberg, S., & Malm, J. R. (1965). Psychiatric complications of open-heart surgery. *New England Journal of Medicine, 273,* 287.

Meyer, B. C., & Blacher, R. S. (1961). A traumatic neurotic reaction induced by succinylcholine chloride. *New York State Journal of Medicine, 61,* 1255–1261.

Rabiner, C. J., & Wilner, A. E. (1980). Differential psychopathological and organic mental disorder at follow-up five years after coronary bypass and cardiac valvular surgery. In H. Speidel & G. Rodewald (Eds.), *Psychic and neurological dysfunctions after open-heart surgery.* (pp. 141–143) New York: Thieme Stratton.

Chapter 9

PSYCHIATRIC PROBLEMS IN OBSTETRIC AND GYNECOLOGIC PATIENTS

Robert O. Pasnau

Many women suffer temporarily or permanently in childhood or in adult age from the fact that they have been born as females.

—Karl Abraham

For many years we have been concerned with psychiatric problems in obstetric and gynecologic patients. Mathis (1967), Golden (1964), Kroger (1962), Norman and Nadelson (1978), Hertz (1974), and many others have observed that what makes obstetrics and gynecology unique is that all the patients are women and that the problems for which they are seeking medical attention are all related to the sexual and reproductive organs. In no other specialty does the clinical work require a physician who understands emotional processes in relationship to reproductive functioning. One of the most challenging problems for the liaison psychiatrist is the fact that most obstetrician-gynecologists do not possess this understanding.

In an earlier report we offered a summary of the most frequently encountered clinical problems for the liaison psychiatrist to obstetrics and gynecology (Pasnau, 1975). These include hospital management problems associated with chronic diseases in pregnancy, assessment of the competency of the mother to care for the infant, postpartum reactions, stillbirth, therapeutic abortion, the unwanted pregnancy, the psychotic pregnant patient, infertility, repeated spontaneous abortions, sterilization, hospital management problems associated with pelvic infection or narcotics addiction, pelvic pain, emotional problems following surgery, menstrual disorders, the dying patient, delirium, and sexual problems. In this chapter we will review briefly some of our past work in several of these areas and then go on to describe some clinical cases that serve to highlight the many issues involved in consultation to obstetric and gynecologic patients.

Twenty years ago we studied patients with amenorrhea who were evaluated for endocrine disorder and psychopathology (Chez, Pasnau, Lecken, & Batiste, 1964). Each was found to have overt endocrine disorder along with a psychiatric diagnosis ranging from neurosis to severe character disorder. Characteristically, the patients had reacted to stress with psychosomatic reactions. On initial examination there was repeated denial of environmental stress or emotional symptoms. Each of the patients underwent a thorough psychiatric and psychologic evaluation. Common denominators were psychosexual immaturity, ambivalence regarding the feminine role, ambivalence about pregnancy, conflicts over heterosexual activity, and general difficulties in interpersonal relationships. Psychologic testing revealed personal isolation and distortion of body image. Three-fourths of women entered psychotherapy; one-fourth declined further psychiatric assistance. Of those who entered psychiatric treatment two-thirds began menstruating spontaneously following or during psychiatric treatment, prior to the treatment of the endocrinologic disorder.

An early area of scientific interest for our group was psychiatric complications of therapeutic abortion (Pasnau, 1972). During the late sixties and early seventies psychiatrists underwent a gradual change of opinion regarding the psychiatric complications of induced abortion. The myth of the serious emotional sequelae was exploded by reevaluation of the older reports and by undertaking new studies. In our new studies most normal women were found to react to abortions with mild feelings of depression without serious aftereffects. Most women who were physically ill were found to respond with improved mental attitudes, although a few were found to respond with increased symptoms. In none of our studies were we able to determine in advance which women would react adversely to pregnancy and which to abortion. We concluded that there was no evidence to suggest that the risk of psychiatric complications in induced abortion constituted a contraindication to the procedure in either normal or psychiatrically ill women.

Nevertheless, we discovered that there were important indications in pre- and postabortion counseling for psychiatric involvement that could not be overlooked. We summarized these as cases in which (a) either the woman exhibited marked ambivalence or the stated motivation for continuing or terminating the pregnancy was suspect; (b) unhealthy, self-destructive, or inappropriate use of sexuality resulted in pregnancy, with the use of abortion as birth control; (c) the woman was incompetent to decide on the continuation or termination of pregnancy; (d) a serious physical illness compromised the ability of the woman to cope emotionally with the issue of pregnancy or abortion; (e) the woman had a history of prior postpartum affective or psychotic illness or prior affective disorder; and (f) the psychiatrist was needed for education of the physician or staff (Marmer, Pasnau, & Cushner, 1974).

We also were involved in a study of the young (under twenty-five), never married, never pregnant women who requested permanent sterilization (Pasnau, 1979). Until recent times many gynecologists had been reluctant to perform tubal ligations on women in this group, fearing that they would be at high risk for dissatisfaction and would probably desire fertility in the future. Yet with the rise of the women's movement and the desire of each woman to decide her reproductive future, many physicians were persuaded to go ahead with the procedure in the face of insufficient data to predict the likelihood of success or failure. We studied a group of these women during a 5-year period. We found that they were generally correct in their surmise that they would in fact not be dissatisfied with the procedure. Many of the patients had histories of maternal deprivation, abuse, or early responsibilities for care of younger siblings. It appeared that they correctly perceived that their adult roles would not be enhanced by assuming the care of children. We concluded that it was very important that these issues be discussed with each patient and that a careful personal history be obtained in each case.

Another study that we conducted was on teenagers requesting therapeutic abortion from a planned parenthood clinic in Los Angeles (Glasser & Pasnau, 1975). We were able to divide the group into several categories, including (a) those young women who, for important psychodynamic reasons, needed to test out their reproductive capacity, (b) those who were poorly educated, (c) those emotionally deprived who, instead of requesting abortion, requested help in keeping their babies, and (d) those who needed to become pregnant in order to convince their parents that they had achieved maturity.

In a separate study of abortion in middle-age women we found that as age at menopause advanced and reproductive years increased, it became increasingly more common for women in their late thirties and forties to request sterilization procedures. Requests for abortions also were more frequently encountered. Ford, Castelnuovo-Tedesco, and Long (1971) showed that older-age women were likely to respond positively to sterilization, particularly those who were multiparous and considered themselves finally freed from their roles as "baby factories." Nonetheless, the procedure is not without problems and conflicts. Abortion in older women, particularly in those who have families, is not without risk. Healthy middle-age women, particularly those with children at home, are more likely to be aware of the significance of their decision to undergo abortion. Whereas younger (teenage) women may experience the abortion process with little or no reflection or anxiety, older women are more likely to reflect on the loss of the fetus and the imagined future of the unborn child and to experience more feelings of grief and regret. This is not to say that such procedures should never be done, only that the physician should be alert to the potential for grief reactions and permit the patient to explore these feelings both before and after the procedure (Farash & Pasnau, 1978).

Another important study carried out by our group focused

on pelvic pain (Pasnau, Soldinger, & Anderson, 1985). As a result of our findings, we have suggested that pelvic pain patients be divided into the following five diagnostic categories:

1. *Patients who have pelvic pathology that explains the pain.* These are patients with positive physical laparoscopic examinations that provide physical explanation of the painful symptoms. Many of these patients may have concomitant psychological problems; for most of these patients the supportive therapy should be provided by the primary care physician while providing the needed physical or medical treatment.

2. *Patients who have pelvic pathology that does not explain the pain.* In this category patients may have a number of physical findings that do not totally explain the painful symptoms. These patients are often observed to be more neurotic or have significantly more emotional problems than those in the first category. For these patients it is essential that the primary care physician take on the role of providing supportive therapy as well as a diagnostic workup. Unfortunately, correcting the underlying medical problem often does not affect the pelvic pain problem to a significant degree.

3. *Patients who have questionable pelvic pain or who have pelvic pathology that may or may not explain the pelvic pain.* These questionable pathologic states have been described as the pelvic congestion syndrome, myofascial or musculoskeletal pain syndromes, changes in pelvic blood flow, difficulty in sexual arousal, vulvar varicosities, and pelvic sympathetic syndromes. This group blends into the one described above, and the implications for treatment and therapy are the same. It is essential that while the workup and the physical symptoms are treated, the primary care physician provide therapeutic and emotional support by establishing a good physician-patient relationship.

4. *Patients who have no discernible pelvic pathology to explain the pelvic pain.* Although this situation rarely exists, when it occurs, such patients are best described as suffering from conversion disorders in which the pelvic pain bears a symbolic relationship to the underlying psychological problem. Occasionally, in either a depressed or psychotic patient the painful symptomatology represents a somatic delusion. Most of the time, however, the underlying pelvic or extrapelvic pathology has not yet been dis-

covered. It is important to continue the evaluation, establishing a positive alliance with the patient and avoiding premature psychiatric referral until the workup is complete.

5. *Chronic pain patients.* These patients have been described as suffering from psychological consequences of pain over a prolonged period of time. They are emotionally disturbed, and the form of the disturbance is usually hypochondriasis and depression. Patients admit that they are preoccupied with their symptoms to the exclusion of almost everything else. They feel quite hopeless about their situation. There is clear evidence that their reaction to chronic pain is not imaginary: it is measurable and seems consistent from patient to patient. For these patients it is not useful to differentiate "psychogenic" pain from "real" pain, because the emotional consequences of pain appear to be independent of the pathology.

Another important study by our group was of psychological reactions to sterilization procedures (Pasnau & Gitlin, 1980). We found that these run the gamut from positive to negative, including normal grief, relief, severe distress, depression, and delayed neurotic reactions. The reactions often were complicated by a lack of physician or family sensitivity and/or support and by the seriousness of the medical problem. Sometimes sterilization became the focus for disability, and the possibility of reversal of the procedure emerged as the focus of the psychiatric inquiry. We found that the role of the liaison psychiatrist was not only to educate the medical team and to raise their awareness to potential problems but also to be sensitive to the patient's emotional needs and provide her with psychiatric treatment whenever appropriate.

Our most recent studies have involved depression in obstetric and gynecologic patients (Gitlin & Pasnau, 1983). This subject, which is plagued by conceptual difficulties, has proved to be very controversial. Two major syndromes in the field, postpartum depression and posthysterectomy depression, may not be distinct illnesses in that they lack consensually validated definitions. Even greater difficulties arise when attempting to evaluate the relationship between premenstrual tension and depression.

The unique problems in evaluating depressive symptoms in

our patients stem from the complex interplay of five separate dimensions:

1. Psychological aspects of sexuality and reproduction make even normal physiologic changes a potential source of emotional vulnerability.

2. Hormonal aspects that involve changes of 100-fold in a matter of days have prompted at least one biological investigator of postpartum depression to suggest that depression is the usual response to such sudden alterations in hormone levels (Gelder, 1978).

3. Problems of symptom and time course variability make syndrome definition and clinical understanding difficult, even if the existence of unique depressive syndromes could be validated.

4. Culturally biased attitudes toward women may have resulted in "the myth of involutional melancholia," which reflected a societal projection of the effect of loss of childbearing capacity on psychiatric functioning even in the absence of scientific data to support it (Weissman, 1979).

5. Prior unrecognized psychopathology may account for a disproportionate number of posthysterectomy and postpartum illnesses.

Nonetheless, three major types of syndromes in obstetrics and gynecologic patients have emerged as more or less accepted clinical entities. These are (a) reactions to loss, (b) postpartum depression and (c) premenstrual tension syndrome. These syndromes have complex clinical pictures with multiple etiologies and contributing factors that range from psychological variables and general stress to hormonal imbalances. Further research in the field should use clearly defined diagnostic criteria and should control for baseline psychopathology. With more rigorous research methodologies much of the present confusion and ignorance that pervades the field of depression in obstetric and gynecologic patients will disappear.

Others in our consultation liaison group have studied problems in human sexuality in obstetrics and gynecologic patients, the problems of the heroin addict and alcoholic patient on the gynecologic service, and cancer in the obstetrics and gynecologic patients (Fawzy & Fawzy, 1982; Wellisch, in press). Hertz (1974) has noted that the overall problems on obstetrics and gynecologic services are similar to those reported by the medical surgical wards. Although this is true, the subjects mentioned above constitute some unique problems in consultation/ liaison psychiatry to obstetrics-gynecology services. In addition, obstetricians and gynecologists have been confronted with more of the important controversial social issues of our time than they are prepared to deal with either by training or interest. This has provided exciting and challenging opportunities for psychiatric involvement in both the training of obstetricians and gynecologists and in consultations with their patients.

In an earlier article we touched on some of the factors that may lead to difficulties in cooperation between the consulting psychiatrist and the obstetrics-gynecology service (Pasnau, 1975). These include the inherent conflict between the illness orientation of the gynecologist and the patient orientation of the psychiatrist. Notman and Nadelson (1978) described their observations during an 18-month period in consultation to obstetrics and gynecology. In their review of 63 consultation reports at the Beth Israel Hospital in Boston, more than 33 percent were on patients presenting psychiatric symptoms about which the physician was concerned or wanted documented. This group included patients with depression, anxiety, bizarre ideation, or documented psychiatric history. For some of these women the consultations contained specific requests for help with management or for information on psychotropic medication. About 25 percent of their patients fell into the category of those who were experiencing emotional reactions to an obstetric or gynecologic experience, including the birth of a defective child, diagnosis of malignancy, or postpartum reactions. In only 1 out of 5 patients were psychiatrists called on to help in the screening or evaluation for a specific procedure, and in only 1 of 10 were they called on for consultation for psychosomatic problems. The latter usually involved patients with pain in whom no physical cause could be found.

To highlight some of these problems we have selected seven recent patients who illustrate some of these challenging clinical problems. These include the management of pregnant chronic schizophrenic women; the treatment of women with bipolar affective disorders who become pregnant during a manic episode; evaluation and treatment of women who experience a postpartum psychosis; management of women who experience an anxiety attack prior to tubal ligation; treatment of women who become depressed following hysterectomy; management of women with "chronic" pelvic infection; and consultation to the women whose mental state deteriorates following cancer therapy. Each of the brief case presentations will be followed by a discussion.

CLINICAL CASES

Case No. 1

The patient was a twenty-three-year-old white female g III, p ō, ab II, who had a 3-year history of bipolar affective disorder age of seventeen. During her first psychiatric hospitalization she was fortunate to have been assigned to a psychiatric resident who agreed to provide continuity of care for the patient during the period of her residency program and to follow the patient after completing her residency. As a result, for the past 8 years the patient has been treated by the same therapist, and the psychiatric history was very complete. The patient was currently living with her mother and her grandmother in a middle-class home. The patient's father, who was diagnosed as schizophrenic, committed suicide when she was five years old. The patient's older brother had been confined in a mental hospital for the past 15 years. Repeated attempts to have the patient treated in a halfway house were resisted by the mother and grandmother on the basis that "we have lost too many family members to schizophrenia." Nonetheless, the family interactions were very difficult for the patient to handle, and the mother was frequently unable to follow through on the suggestions made by the psychiatrist for specific management of the patient. The patient had been on high doses of Prolixin® for the past 5 years and had been seen weekly in outpatient therapy.

She had no idea how she became pregnant, and the therapist was surprised when she learned of the pregnancy because she had been unaware that the patient had had sexual contacts, although the patient has had many sexual fantasies and delusions over the 8-year period. It was not discovered that she was pregnant until well into the second trimester when the mother had the patient examined by a gynecologist. The patient did not wish to have an abortion, and the mother and grandmother expressed an interest in raising the child in an attempt to replace family members who had been previously lost to illness. The patient was admitted to a psychiatric hospital for evaluation of her mental state, discontinuing her medications, and for developing a plan to manage the patient during pregnancy and labor and for planning for the future of the infant.

The plight of the schizophrenic woman who becomes pregnant and delivers a child is sensitively described in the recent Broadway play *Agnes of God*, in which a psychotic woman delivers her baby and murders it because it is "a mistake." This highlights the fact that a primary concern for the psychiatrist is the welfare of the baby in addition to the welfare of the mother. The primary clinical point is that whenever and at whatever trimester the pregnancy is discovered, the patient should be hospitalized and all psychotropic medications discontinued. Even though the time of greatest teratogenic vulnerability is in the first trimester, there is increasing evidence to indicate that the effects of the neuroleptic agents may affect fetal and newborn brain development (Ameer, 1979). It has now been shown that even small doses of phenobarbital may have an adverse effect on the infant's further development (Heinonen, Sloane, & Shapiro, 1977). Therefore, all such medication should be stopped for the duration of the pregnancy.

Interestingly, many pregnant chronic psychotic patients do extremely well during their pregnancy. Perhaps because the high levels of hormones have an antipsychotic effect, some schizophrenic women experience a remission (Sandler, 1978). This has led to the speculation that schizophrenic women may become repeatedly pregnant in order to experience the antipsychotic effect of such pregnancies. The public health considerations include raising the level of potentially psychotic individuals in the genetic pool, as well as great problems in providing adequate protection for the infants of these mothers. It also requires special liaison with the obstetrics department in order to provide good transition between the services when the patient is referred for labor and delivery. Such patients should be encouraged to attend La Maze classes with a family member to help them prepare for labor and delivery, and the physician should be alerted to special problems that may exist during the course of the labor period. In our hospital, social workers have provided important links to necessary community agencies and have provided great support to families of such patients. In the case of the patient described above, medications were stopped, the patient experienced a remission, and she was able to be discharged from the hospital to be followed at home by her psychiatrist until delivery.

Case No. 2

The patient was a twenty-three-year-old white female g Ⅲ, p ō, ab Ⅱ, who had a 3-year history of bipolar affective disorder with a positive family history. Her father, who was a banker, had a long history of manic-depressive illness and successful lithium treatment. The patient, however, had been unsuccessfully controlled due to noncompliance and poor judgment. During each of her three episodes of mania she became involved in unprotected sexual activity and subsequently became pregnant. Because of poor judgment she did not seek psychiatric treatment and required involuntary hospitalization on each of these occasions. On each of the previous occasions it was possible to treat her with antipsychotic agents, secure her permission for a therapeutic abortion, and terminate the pregnancy. During her last hospitalization, though she was psychotic and delusional, the patient claimed that she wished to continue the pregnancy and have the baby. Because her private psychiatrist was disinclined to use any antipsychotic medication or lithium in view of the patient's desire to continue her pregnancy, she was committed to the UCLA Neuropsychiatric Institute involuntarily for evaluation and management of her manic episode.

This case involves many important points, including some

medical-legal considerations. In view of recent court decisions it was prudent for the referring psychiatrist to refer the patient for hospitalization and not to use antipsychotic medication. If the psychiatrist had employed the antipsychotic medication and the fetus had become impaired, there is legal precedent for suit against the psychiatrist on behalf of the child for malpractice years later (W. Winslade, personal communication, 1982). On the other hand, the patient was a clear danger to herself (and possibly to her unborn fetus) as a result of her psychosis and impaired judgment. The family problems were intense. The father insisted that the patient be hospitalized and the pregnancy terminated. In this case the patient was admitted to the hospital and given an intravenous injection of droperidol (a very rapidly excreted antipsychotic agent), and she responded almost immediately. Within 4 h she was discussing her problems rationally; she agreed to have a therapeutic abortion and asked for assistance from her family. At that time it was possible to do an adequate family assessment, develop a treatment plan, and arrange for the abortion. Two days following the abortion the patient signed herself out of the hospital, refusing further medication or psychiatric treatment. At last report she had depleted her funds and appeared to be entering a depressed phase of her illness.

The use of droperidol, while obviously not without risk, is useful in such cases because the impact on fetal circulation is minimal, and its intravenous use permits a very rapid antipsychotic effect.

Case No. 3

The patient was a thirty-year-old g ī, p ī, ab ō white female who delivered twin boys by cesarean section. Her parents were both survivors of Nazi persecution. The children were named after the patient's siblings who had died in a German concentration camp. Three days following her delivery the patient began experiencing severe feelings of depression, agitation, and fantasies of killing her babies. She did not tell anyone of these fantasies, however, and it was only on her return home that she was noted to be inattentive to her children, distracted, and showing severe psychomotor retardation. Her husband, who did not understand his wife's reaction, called his in-laws, who berated the patient for her ingratitude for the privilege of having children and living in a free country. Shortly following this she made a serious suicide attempt by swallowing a number of sleeping capsules. She was admitted to the Neuropsychiatric Institute with a diagnosis of postpartum depression. On admission she appeared to be depressed and delusional. She believed that the ward attendants were concentration camp guards, and she spoke in a mixture of Polish, German, Yiddish, and English. Her course was marked by very gradual progress. She was treated with antipsychotic medication, and on no response to that she was changed to antidepressant medication. Eventually, she was placed on lithium carbonate. Psychotherapy was extremely difficult, and there was little family cooperation with her treatment. However, after 6 weeks of intensive treatment she was able to return home on a home visit, where she was able to interact with her husband and her children. Her symptoms gradually subsided, and she was treated with a combination of tricyclic antidepressants and lithium carbonate.

From the time of Hippocrates, it has been observed that certain women experience rather severe postpartum reactions, ranging from delirium to severe depression. Even though there are many methodological problems in the research, especially in the definition of depression, it is now agreed that three depressive syndromes exist in the postpartum period:

1. Postpartum "blues," characterized as a mild disturbance that is seen within the first 10 days following delivery
2. Severe psychotic depression, which is a more uncommon syndrome, occurring primarily between the third and fourteenth postpartum day
3. Moderate depression, which is a depressive syndrome that is apparently indistinguishable from major affective disorder (Gitlin & Pasnau, 1983)

Postpartum blues occur in a majority of women, probably between 50 and 80 percent. A recent report showed that 76 percent of East African women demonstrate a mild postpartum mood disturbance, indicating that this disorder crosses cultural boundaries (Harris, 1981). These blues typically begin during the first week postpartum. A hormonal etiology is suspected. However, the most meaningful study of postpartum blues has shown that there are no hormonal differences between those women experiencing the blues and those not experiencing them. Risk factors include the primiparous pregnancy, a history of premenstrual tension, and no obstetric variables. The disorder is self-limiting and usually requires no specific treatment other than reassurance. A small minority progress to develop a severe depressive illness.

Severe postpartum psychosis is relatively uncommon, although confusion, emotional lability, and agitation are common in postpartum depression. These postpartum psychotic disorders are characterized by significant psychosis, emotional labilty, and disorientation and often are seen in women who have undergone cesarean section. Whether these postoperative delirium patients should be categorized with postpartum reactions is not clear. The incidence of postpartum psychosis is approximately 1 in 50 births. Four-fifths of these are psychotic depressions. The variables associated with this disorder are (a) primiparous status, (b) unmarried status, (c) cesarean birth, and (d) past history of psychiatric disorder. Women who have a history of postpartum disorders have a 30 percent risk history of manic-depressive illness. With respect to treatment and prognosis, severe postpartum depression is similar to that of non-postpartum depression—i.e., recovery rates are high and generally extend to full remissions. However, occasional patients present very recalcitrant and resistant symptoms, and the treatment may be difficult and prolonged.

There is also an increased risk for moderate depression in the first month to 2 years following delivery. These disorders are typically ones that blur with the mild blues, as well as a more severe hospitalized depression. The primary symptoms are affective lability, tearfulness, insomnia, and agitation, which last for weeks to months. Between 3 and 20 percent of all postpartum women manifest a moderate depression syndrome within 1 year following delivery. These disorders tend to be related to stresses during the pregnancy and to premorbid personality disorders. These may be women who are at risk for development of depression in relationship to stress. Both anxiety and depression during pregnancy seem to correlate with moderate postpartum depression.

In summary, there is a marked increase in the incidence of depression in the postpartum period both immediately and for up to 2 years. The depressions range from mild and transient to severe and disruptive illnesses. Although there are probably clinical differences between postpartum depression and other kinds of depression, the similarities are far more striking and treatment should follow the usual clinical guidelines.

Case No. 4

The patient was a thirty-nine-year-old woman who had been married for 20 years and who had not become pregnant during her marriage. She separated from her husband and on consulting her physician about contraceptives was told that there was "no guarantee" that she could not become pregnant with a new sexual partner. After several weeks of anxiety and ambivalence she consulted her physician to request a tubal ligation sterilization. She decided on this because she and her sexual partner were desirous of engaging in sexual activity without fear of unwanted pregnancy, and both of them found most methods of birth control unacceptable.

On admission to the hospital she found herself unaccountably sad. The night before her surgery she began crying and could not stop. Her physician became alarmed, and she requested psychiatric consultation. In a discussion of the situation with the patient, it appeared that her motivation was sound and that her ambivalence was understandable in relationship to a potential loss that she was quite capable of understanding. The following day she underwent the surgery without difficulty, and she experienced no adverse sequelae. She was seen in follow-up psychiatric consultation; it was apparent that she had adjusted well to the sterilization and was actively involved in planning her future life.

This patient underscores the fact that any decision regarding fertility involves considerable emotional consequence and that no decision for sterilization is made without some degree of ambivalence. Nevertheless, the presence of sad affect should not deter the physician; it merely confirms the observation that fertility is one of the most psychologically charged areas for all women.

It is important to counsel women who are seeking tubal ligation. The major problem is in helping the patient make an informed decision and in allowing time for the process to be worked through. Usually, there is sufficient time for decision-making for sterilization procedures (as opposed to the limited time available to those in abortion counseling). Many women who elect to undergo tubal ligation change their minds after several weeks. Delay in this decision is indicated, considering the usual irreversibility of this procedure.

However, it is also important to note that sterilization procedures appear to be followed by fewer psychological problems than hysterectomy. Most studies indicate that women undergoing tubal ligation have few or no psychiatric sequelae. In one study, for example, only 3 percent of the women had constant regret, and only 21 percent had occasional regrets following tubal ligation (Enoch & Johnes, 1975).

Occasional adverse reactions do occur. These reactions include normal grief, severe distress, depression, and delayed neurotic reactions, as we noted earlier (Pasnau & Gitlin, 1980).

Case No. 5

This patient was a forty-seven-year-old white female, g v̄, p v̄, ab ō, married to a college professor. She underwent hysterectomy for a severe menometrorrhagia secondary to uterine fibroids. She had an uneventful surgery, but during the discussion with her physician following her postoperative checkup she was told that the operation sometimes interferes with sexual functioning and that she should make an effort to "seduce" her husband as soon as she felt like it in order that their sexual life might not suffer. She dated the onset of her depressed mood from this discussion. She became unable to sleep or eat and gradually withdrew from all social involvements. She began to lose weight, was unable to concentrate, and was afraid that she was losing her mind because her memory became so impaired. She was referred for psychiatric consultation by her gynecologist with a diagnosis of posthysterectomy syndrome.

The patient was seen in psychiatric evaluation, placed on a tricyclic antidepressant, and followed for 1 year in weekly psychotherapy sessions. During this time many of her family problems were explored, and as she improved, her husband's behavior deteriorated. He became more alcoholic, became involved with other women, and eventually left the patient and his five children. It appeared to the patient that her surgery had precipitated a family crisis that had resulted not only in her own personal changes but also in an upset in the equilibrium in her family, which she came to recognize as "probably inevitable."

The loss of any internal organ or biological capacity usually provokes a mourning period. These reactions are particularly intense for sexual organs because of the strong associations with gender identity. More than 40 years ago Lindemann (1941) suggested that pelvic surgery provoked disproportionate postoperative disturbances. The most frequent problem in reviewing the literature is in the use of the term *depression,* which is used to refer to a number of nonspecific disorders including reports of feeling depressed. Because of this problem in definition, estimates of posthysterectomy depression vary widely from 6 percent in one study to 70 percent. Other studies have not supported these conclusions. The typical posthysterectomy syndrome is characterized by hot flushes, fatigue, headaches, insomnia, and dizziness, as well as depressed mood. The symptoms often exist without depression and are often found in patients who meet the criteria for a diagnosis of Briquet's syndrome. The highest-risk patients include those with preoperative history of depression and marital disruption. Other risk factors include a lack of demonstrable pelvic pathology (Martin, Roberts, & Clayton, 1980).

Given the paucity of our knowledge regarding the characteristics of posthysterectomy depressive syndrome, it is not surprising that there are few clues to its etiology. Hormonal causes are possible, but no evidence points in that direction. The fact that the peak incidence of referral occurs 2 years after surgery and that there is an increased incidence of psychiatric disorder in patients with marital disruption certainly suggests that psychodynamic factors may be the most significant ones in the etiology of this disorder.

Our own clinical experience supports the importance of psychodynamic factors. Most of the women whom we have seen in consultation for posthysterectomy syndrome have been those with rather serious marital or family disruptions, in which the psychotherapeutic intervention has been the major factor. In any case the diagnosis of "involutional melancholia" has been removed from the psychiatric nomenclature because of the lack of evidence of increased incidence or prevalence of depression in the age range of forty-five to fifty-five, presumably the most common decade for the biological menopause (Weissman, 1979). Thus, although psychological issues that may stem from the symbolic loss of childbearing capacity, as well as psychosocial variables common in this age group, exist, no evidence suggests a specific depressive syndrome in the menopausal period.

Case No. 6

The patient was a twenty-six-year-old, g ō, p ō, ab ō, white female who had been admitted the preceding evening with a pelvic inflammatory disease. The patient had abused the staff both physically and verbally, complaining that only one nurse really understood her problem. She pulled out her intravenous needle, knocked charts off the desk of the nursing station, and generally created havoc. It was the opinion of the head nurse on the unit that she should be transferred to the psychiatry service. From her medical record it was learned that she had been admitted on 12 previous occasions with recurrent salpingitis and on at least 10 of those occasions had been seen by a liaison psychiatrist. On two occasions she had been transferred to the psychiatric unit, where she was diagnosed as having a borderline personality disorder. Previous psychiatric evaluations had revealed a history of multiple foster homes, child abuse, and considerable psychologic deprivation. She had a very stormy relationship with her alcoholic mother, who had appeared intoxicated in the hospital on several occasions. On this occasion the liaison psychiatrist decided not to see the patient; instead he convened a meeting of the health care team (gynecology residents, attending physicians, head nurse, and nurses) to discuss the problems of a patient with emotional difficulties who had a recurrent problem. Several of these nurses expressed feelings that a sexually promiscuous patient such as this, who brought on her own problems, did not deserve modern medical attention. Other staff members felt that the patient was psychotic and that the proper place for her was in a psychiatric unit. Eventually, it was agreed that the patient should receive the best medical attention possible, provided that her antisocial and disruptive behavior could be controlled. A behavioral treatment plan was instituted, and a psychiatrist who had seen her on a previous admission was consulted. With the help of the older psychiatrist and the renewed cooperation of the staff, the patient's symptoms gradually subsided. The patient was followed up in the psychiatric outpatient clinic. She had not been readmitted to the gynecology service with a recurrent pelvic infection.

There are some patients whose entry into the hospital immediately triggers hostile reactions and defensive negativity on the part of the staff. This behavior is often seen in the cases of narcotic addicts, those who have made suicide attempts, and those whose careless or self-inflicted injury has caused their hospitalization. On the gynecology service these are often patients with recurrent pelvic inflammatory disease. Usually these patients are also narcotic addicts, women engaged in prostitution, and/or women who have venereal infections. Their behavior almost always provokes the nursing staff into negative or defensive withdrawal. These patients are described as having borderline personalities. If the illness is trivial or minor, the personality problems rarely matter. However, in the case of serious or life-threatening situations the disruptive behavior may represent a suicidal potential or threaten the continuation of the health care system. Psychiatric treatment rarely benefits such disturbed individuals. However, some behavioral treatment is necessary so the staff can manage the patient's behavior without reacting in despair, acting punitively, or disrupting the future relationship with the medical profession. These patients cause some of the most difficult problems for liaison psychiatrists (Graves, 1975). In fact, the psychiatrist's reputation is often at stake when such patients are referred for consultation. The key factor is the importance of working with the staff to develop a behavioral plan to control the disruptive behavior of the patient and prevent untimely expulsion from the hospital.

Case No. 7

The patient was a seventy-year-old g ī ī p ī ī ab ō, white female with a four-year history of ovarian carcinoma. She had previously undergone total abdominal hysterectomy and bilateral oophorectomy followed by a variety of radiation and chemical therapies for cancer. Following this treatment she had been in good health for 2 years until she was admitted for a recurrence of cancer that appeared to be widespread throughout her peritoneum. Brain scan revealed some brain metastases, and she was begun on a treatment regimen that included the administration of intrathecal methotrexate. During the hospitalization, her forty-year-old daughter was frequently in attendance, often complaining about her mother's care and requesting that her mother be made more comfortable, either with pain medication, antianxiety agents, or antidepressant medication. On rounds the patient frequently was observed crying and eventually was referred for psychiatric consultation to rule out depressive disorder. At the time of the consultation it was observed that the patient was showing considerable emotional lability. She seemed confused as to the date and time of day and occasionally appeared to be disoriented as to place. Nonetheless, she was an extremely bright and intelligent woman who was aware of her fluctuating mental state and extremely distracted and distressed by her mental deterioration. She was also frightened by the insistence of the staff that she "eat." She interpreted her weight loss and their preoccupation with her nutrition as indication that she was dying. She revealed that after 45 years of marriage her husband, who was an attorney, had divorced her 1 year before her cancer was diagnosed and had married a much younger and more attractive woman. Shortly before the consultation her ex-husband had visited her in the hospital and told her, "I'll see you at the River Styx." She was also very upset that her son was being married on the next weekend, and she would not be present for the wedding. Although she claimed to be reassured by her daughter's presence, she recognized that her daughter's anxiety was causing considerable difficulties for the staff.

The primary treatment efforts were directed toward the patient's daughter in an attempt to help her deal more realistically with the recurrence of her mother's illness and with the staff, who had developed considerable identification with the patient and sadness over the inevitable and relentless course of her illness. The son and his new wife visited their mother shortly before her death, and she became much more comfortable as the staff became less insistent on her performance of certain behaviors and more accepting of her coping efforts and her periodic organic brain syndrome.

This case was very complicated, and it raises many important clinical issues. It has been observed that the most frequent cause of organic brain syndrome in oncology patients is the use of intrathecal methotrexate for cerebral metastases. Often such patients are delirious and emotionally labile, and they are confused with patients with depression. At the same time there are problems associated with the recurrence, the family distress and dislocations, and the inevitable recognition by the patient of the exacerbation. The patient's distress leads in turn to considerable psychosocial distress in the health care team and the family. Obviously, such problems are similar to those encountered in medical or surgical oncology. The need to care for the family, the special role the psychiatric consultant can play with the family in mourning, and the techniques of working with the dying patient have all been emphasized in recent publications (Wahl, in press). Yet the role of the consultant to the staff that treats these patients requires special attention in gynecologic oncology. Part of the problem unique to gynecology is the benign setting of the ward milieu. Here patients are not supposed to die but are supposed to become well and leave the hospital. Even though there are a few acute situations in which patients do die unexpectedly, little time is spent with these women prior to their deaths, and the staff experience little of the grief or sadness so common to the staffs of medical or surgical cancer units. Thus, when faced with only a few cancer patients on their ward, the staff may be less well prepared emotionally to deal with them. In such cases, in which the physicians and staff are faced with the sense of loss and sadness, the psychiatric consultant can do much to insure that the patient does not die alone (Wahl, in press).

Table 9-1. Five-Year Summary of the Most Frequently Encountered Clinical Problems in Psychiatric Liaison to Obstetrics-Gynecology

OBSTETRICS
1. Hospital management problems associated with chronic diseases and pregnancy, including
   - A. diabetes
   - B. hypertension
   - C. sickle cell anemia
   - D. toxemia
   - E. personality disorder
   - F. psychosis
2. Assessment of the competency of mother to care for the infant
3. Postpartum reactions: psychosis, depression
4. Stillbirth
5. The unwanted pregnancy—Therapeutic abortion
6. The psychotic patient in labor
7. Infertility
8. Repeated spontaneous abortions
9. Sterilization: family planning clinic problems
10. Problems related to father's presence in delivery room

GYNECOLOGY
1. Hospital management problems associated with
   - A. pelvic infection
   - B. narcotics addiction
   - C. personality disorder
   - D. psychosis
2. Pelvic pain, including dyspareunia, dysmenorrhea
3. Emotional reactions following pelvic surgery
4. Menstrual disorder, including menopausal syndromes
5. The dying patient and her family
6. Delirium
7. Sexual counseling

SUMMARY AND CONCLUSION

The varied clinical problems that confront the psychiatric consultant in obstetrics and gynecology, although not unique to this subspeciality, are complex and challenging. We have tried to present issues that are highlighted by obstetrics and gynecologic patients. In all of these situations skillful handling of sensitive issues is required with patients, families, physicians, and staff. And for all of these problems the psychiatrist as consultant must be well versed in all aspects of psychiatric treatment, behavioral medicine, and psychopharmacology. The psychiatrist must be identified as someone who has the interest and expertise to solve the behavioral or psychiatric problems. Our experiences in obstetrics and gynecology attest to the need for liaison psychiatric involvement and to the very great opportunity that exists in this area for service, education, and research.

REFERENCES

Ameer, B. (1979). Teratology of psychoactive drugs. In J. M. Davis & D. Greenblatt (Eds.), *Psychopharmacology update: New and neglected areas*. (pp. 1-14) New York; Grune & Stratton.

Chez, R., Pasnau, R. O., Lecken, S., & Batiste, C. (1964). Psychiatric aspects of acquired amenorrhea. *Obstetrics and Gynecology, 24,* 549–553.

Enoch, M. D., & Johnes, K. (1975). Sterilization: A review of 98 sterilized women. *British Journal of Psychiatry, 127,* 583–587.

Farash, J., & Pasnau, R. O. (1978). Loss and amniocentesis abortion. In C. Hollingsworth & R. O. Pasnau (Eds.), *The family in mourning.* New York: Grune & Stratton.

Fawzy, F. I., & Fawzy, N. (1982). Psychosocial aspects of cancer. In D. W. Nixon (Ed.), *Diagnosis and management of cancer*. (pp. 111-123) Menlo Park, CA: Addison-Wesley.

Ford, C., Castelnuovo-Tedesco, P., & Long, K. (1971). Is abortion a therapeutic procedure in psychiatry? *Journal of the American Medical Association, 213,* 1173–1178.

Gelder, M. G. (1978). Hormones in post partum depression. In M.

Sandler (Ed.), *Mental illness in pregnancy and the puerperium.* Oxford: Oxford University Press.

Gitlin, M. J., & Pasnau, R. O. (1983). Depression in obstetric and gynecology patients. *Journal of Psychiatric Treatment Evaluation, 5,* 421–428.

Glasser, M., & Pasnau, R. O. (1975). The unwanted pregnancy in adolescence. *Journal of Family Practice, 2,* 91–94.

Golden, J. S. (1964). Psychosomatic problems in obstetric and gynecologic practice. In C. W. Wahl (Ed.), *New dimensions in psychosomatic medicine.* (pp. 97–115) Boston: Little, Brown.

Graves, J. (1975). Management of the borderline patient on a medical-surgical ward: The psychiatric consultant's role. *International Journal of Psychiatry Medicine, 6,* 337–348.

Harris, B. (1981). Maternity blues in East African clinic attenders. *Archives of General Psychiatry, 38,* 1293–1295.

Heinonen, O. P., Sloane, D., & Shapiro, S. (1977). *Birth defects and drugs in pregnancy.* Littleton, MA: Publishing Science Group.

Hertz, D. G. (1974). Problems and challenges of consultation-psychiatry in obstetrics-gynecology. *Psychotherapy and Psychosomatics, 23,* 67–77.

Kroger, W. (1962). *Psychosomatic obstetrics, gynecology, and endocrinology.* Springfield, IL: Charles C. Thomas.

Lindemann, E. (1941–42). Observations on psychiatric sequelae to surgical operations in women. *American Journal of Psychiatry, 98,* 132–139.

Marmer, S. S., Pasnau, R. O., & Cushner, I. M. (1974). Is psychiatric consultation in abortion obsolete? *International Journal of Psychiatry Medicine, 5,* 201–209.

Martin, R. L., Roberts, W. V., & Clayton, P. J. (1980). Psychiatric status after hysterectomy. *Journal of the American Medical Association, 244,* 350–353.

Mathis, J. (1967). Psychiatry and the obstetrician-gynecologist. *Medical Clinics of North America, 51,* 1375–1380.

Notman, M. T., & Nadelson, C. C. (1978). *The woman patient: Medical and psychological interfaces.* New York: Plenum Press.

Pasnau, R. O. (1972). Psychiatric complications of therapeutic abortion. *Obstetrics and Gynecology, 40,* 252–256.

Pasnau, R. O. (1975). Psychiatry and obstetrics-gynecology: Report of a five-year experience in psychiatric liaison. In R. O. Pasnau (Ed.), *Consultation liaison psychiatry.* New York: Grune & Stratton.

Pasnau, R. O. (1979). Psychiatric consultation for obstetric and gynecologic patients. *Psychiatry Digest, 40,* 25–30.

Pasnau, R. O., & Gitlin, J. J. (1980). Psychological reactions to sterilization procedures. *Psychosomatics, 21,* 10–14.

Pasnau, R. O., Soldinger, S., & Anderson, B. L. (1985). Pelvic pain. In R. G. Priest (Ed.), *Psychiatric disorders in obstetrics and gynecology:* London: Butterworth.

Sandler, M. (1978). *Mental illness in pregnancy and the puerperium.* New York: Oxford University Press.

Wahl, C. W. (in press). Helping the dying patient and family. In R. O. Pasnau (Ed.), *Psychosocial aspects of medical practice: Vol. 2. Adults and the elderly.* Menlo Park, CA: Addison-Wesley.

Weissman, M. M. (1979). The myth of involutional melancholia. *Journal of the American Medical Association, 242,* 247.

Wellisch, D. I. (in press). Psychological aspects of the medical treatment of the heroin addict. In R. O. Pasnau (Ed.), *Psychosocial aspects of medical practice: Vol. 2. Adults and elderly.* Menlo Park, CA: Addison-Wesley.

PART III

CHRONIC ILLNESS

Chapter 10

PARKINSON'S DISEASE: LIVING WITH UNCERTAINTY

Hilde Bruch

I appreciate the opportunity to report my own experiences with Parkinson's disease, which befell me about 10 years ago. I chose the subtitle "Living with Uncertainty" because I feel that the unpredictability of forever changing symptoms is the hardest aspect to accept. To give just one example, I am never certain whether I will stay controlled or whether I will suffer from tremor during a talk, whether my voice will be clear or shaky.

The illness was described by Parkinson in 1817 as "shaking palsy," with tremor, muscular rigidity, and slowness of bodily movements as the main symptoms. The onset is gradual, often so slow that the first symptoms are apt to be overlooked. I first noticed a peculiar pain in my right thigh, which I attributed to the pin inserted 2 years earlier for a broken hip. Everything was all right with the hip, but the difficulties in walking persisted, and I noticed some tremor in my right hand. For at least 6 to 8 years the symptoms were strictly limited to the right side of the body and disappeared during sleep.

I was sixty-nine years old when I consulted Dr. Ben Cooper, and the symptoms were so mild that the possibility of my suffering from familial tremor was considered. About 2 months later the diagnosis of Parkinson's disease was made. As time went on, I did not find it easy to separate signs of aging from the spreading symptoms of parkinsonism. I must admit that I was not prepared for the symptomatology of either. I had never known anyone with parkinsonism. A 3-years-younger sister and I are the only survivors of a once large family in which nobody else lived to be seventy. Thus, I had no model or knowledge of what happens to people and how they change with advancing years, and how they deal with an unknown disease.

As far as I remember, my emotional reaction to the fact of having parkinsonism was amazingly mild, practically a denial of illness. I had a somewhat facetious reaction, that it was a case of ironic justice that this illness with the incessant movements had happened to me, who had a lifelong record of avoiding muscular activities. I had enjoyed some sports, such as swimming, skiing, and horseback riding, but I utterly disliked anything that smelled of calisthenics or "exercise."

I knew so little about Parkinsonism that my first reaction was a kind of relief. If I had to have an illness with advancing years, then Parkinsonism looked to me like a rather limited disease. All one had to do was compensate for a certain shakiness and be doubly careful in handling breakable objects. What I was not prepared for was that this illness affects one's whole range of activities, everything that one does in a 24-h cycle of living.

What puzzles me now in retrospect is that I showed so little curiosity to find out something about this illness. I knew in a vague way that there had been an operation during the sixties and that since that time the connection with dopamine had been discovered; and I felt lucky in a way that there was medication that could control the symptoms. In 1978 I read and found helpful a guide (Duvoisin, 1978) for patients and families. More recently I read *Parkinson's: A Patient's View* (Dorros, 1981).

At first my nights were undisturbed; if anything, I slept better than before. The first handicaps were related to dressing and cooking. The difficulties increased gradually, but I soon noticed that holding a lightweight article provoked more shaking. The greatest difficulty was how to put on stockings. For the first few years I considered such handicaps challenges to my ingenuity, and I avoided movements that would lead to shaking.

Gradually, 6 to 8 years later, loss of muscle coordination became handicapping. I had always enjoyed swimming, and I spent the summer of 1977 with my sister, who had access to an Olympic-size swimming pool. I had planned to practice and increase my endurance and was quite pleased with my progress, when suddenly I could not coordinate my arms and legs. Since then I have made several efforts to resume swimming but without success.

Poor coordination made itself felt in several ways; most dangerous is a tendency to stumble and fall. In November 1980 I fell entering the library building and broke my left hip. I was taken to an emergency room, and there a difficult situation developed. I had taken my medication at lunchtime and fell on the way back to my office. After several hours in the emergency room I began shaking and needed another dose of medication. However, the surgeon had left an order to keep me from eating and drinking. I finally swallowed some tablets without water; I was afraid I would fall off the stretcher.

After the broken hip I accepted walking with a cane. But there are always short walks where one cannot use a cane. In May 1982 I fell right in my living room when getting out of a chair; I nearly fell against the television set, ending up behind it with a broken left arm. The hardest difficulty was reaching a telephone to ask for help.

I had always enjoyed cooking and felt I could continue with it, though it meant simplification in many areas, such as using one set of dishes instead of changing them around, emphasis on broiled foods, even using prepared food. The changes ocurred over a long period of time, and I felt I was lucky that I could handle knife and fork properly; difficulties with that became apparent only during the last few years.

As I recall it, the progression of symptoms took place gradually, rarely as suddenly as the difficulties with swimming. I learned to compensate for each difficulty or to ask for help. I might describe what went on during the first 6 or 8 years as a growing awkwardness in doing accustomed things, such as fastening my watchband or the clasp of a necklace, or writing legibly. All of these things were annoying, but none was big enough to interfere with the cycle of my activities. I relate the very limited extent of emotional reaction to having Parkinson-ism to a lifelong habit of remaining calm and unemotional in the face of difficulties. I did not look far beyond the immediate symptoms.

I learned very gradually that Parkinson's disease affects the whole person, and my self-image changed. Having considered myself a calm person with a high threshold for reacting to worry or emotional upset, I learned now that I reacted emotionally much more often and more strongly than I had been aware of. Parkinsonism acted like an amplifier of mild responses, which suddenly became noticeable through the shaking they pro-voked. One of my first observations was that when driving, the right hand began to tremble when there was the slightest ques-tion, like "At what exit do I leave the highway?" It was a rela-tively mild disturbance as long as it was restricted to my hand, but it became a sign of some danger when the right foot on the pedal started to shake. I adjusted to these things by not driving at night or when it rained and by avoiding freeways and main traffic streets.

Gradually, I noticed that I reacted with shaking whenever there was the slightest experience of uncertainty. It became a major issue when I was being kept waiting and I felt helpless and abandoned in the situation. No amount of argument with my-self changed the extent of my shaking, which was particularly severe when I feared being late. I also noted that I was much more often annoyed or anxious, usually to a mild degree, than I would have noticed or reacted to in the past. The only reason I "knew" I was under stress was the more severe tremor.

I was mildly amused by the selectivity of feeling embar-rassed or upset. On the whole I didn't mind undergoing changes in my outer appearance. I was aware of children reacting in different ways. A great-niece living in England, age five or six at the time, was greatly alarmed when my hand started to shake; she held it to quiet it down and shouted, "Stop it, stop it." In contrast, a great-nephew who knew me well reacted with help-ful concern: "I'll help you up the stairs."

I myself am impressed by the definite distinction I make among various changes. I feel very uneasy about the paucity of facial expressions, about looking like a "poker face" or somewhat annoyed or uninvolved. I accepted the stooping forward and a certain clumsiness of walking quite readily but felt very uneasy about becoming shorter and also lighter in weight. Throughout life I had thought of myself as a big person, and the diminished body image still sounds quite unrealistic to me.

As I mentioned before, the increase of symptoms was gradual, but during the last 3 years they have been increasing, and the effectiveness of medication appears diminished. At around that time a new secretary came to work for me, and she made a number of pertinent observations. She wrote them out, and I quote from the remarks of Mrs. Shirley Hoston:

> When I came to work in late November 1979 there were some obvious effects of Parkinsonism and of age in general: the posture, occasional shaking of the hand (particularly when holding a piece of paper or something else lightweight, or when upset). Yet she did most things for herself, getting what was needed from files, handling papers and paper clips, using the dictating machine, etc. Outside the office she drove, walked to lunch nearly every day, didn't mention any problems with shopping, dressing, and cooking. I was surprised to realize that she thought of herself as a physically large person (and that she had in fact been considerably taller and heavier a few years earlier). I felt much bigger as well as stronger than her.
>
> Whatever changes came about in the first year I can't distinctly recall; they must have been small and gradual. I became more involved at the time of the broken hip in November 1980. It may be hard to separate the hip-related "neediness" from the Parkinson-related disability. In general I might say the hip caused few problems after a very short time, yet there were more and more things with which she needed help.

Then comes an enumeration of various things, such as dropping papers when I had to sort them out, being unable to affix paper clips or to take a letter out of its envelope, difficulties with writing, getting dressed, and driving the car.

REACTION TO MEDICATION

My overall attitude has been and continues to be one of gratitude that the illness did not befall me until after L-dopa had become available. I received several medications in slightly varying amounts: from 1973 to 1976, L-dopa; from 1976 to 1978, carbidopa with L-dopa, and amantadine. Since November 1981 I have been part of a research project to test the effectiveness of a new drug, at times in combination with ethopropazine hydrochloride and diphenhydramine hydrochloride.

I was impressed by the effectiveness of L-dopa in stopping the shaking and rigidity. The great difficulty was its strong effect on the vomiting center. I reacted with nausea from the very beginning, and it did not seem to improve with the change to the carbidopa/L-dopa combination, which I could take only in relatively small doses. The vomiting could be controlled by eating something within a 20-min period. This became a difficulty when traveling. It was always the same dilemma: without medication I could not get dressed, and breakfast was not always served soon enough. I got into the habit of carrying bread sticks in my pocketbook, which even in moderate quantity protected against the vomiting impulse.

Except for the effect on the nausea center I enjoyed taking L-dopa; I have a definite feeling that it has an "up" effect. I had the same feeling about the combination of L-dopa with carbidopa—that it improved my mood, even my energy level.

I am afraid that my memory for the various reactions to the illness is rather poor. But judging from the amount of traveling, I was still quite active during the first 6 or 8 years. In 1975 I went to Australia and New Zealand with an American Psychiatric Association group. I do not remember any difficulties with medication or with Parkinson symptoms, except for one incident. On the plane from Houston to Los Angeles I ordered a cocktail and took the pills that were due at that time, expecting that some snack would be served. Unfortunately nothing was served, and when the meal tray came the delay had been too long and I upchucked my meal. This is the only memory of a mishap on the 3-week trip.

My reaction to the medication was positive, and I attribute my not having become depressed, even for a short period, while facing the steadily increasing handicaps of the Parkinson's condition to the medication. From 1979 on I took amantadine to better control the shaking, continuing carbidopa with L-dopa in rather small doses. I firmly believe that amantadine protected me against the flu and other infections. The simple fact is that I had amazingly few infections while suffering from Parkinsonism—with one exception, namely, a severe reaction to a smallpox inoculation July 1974. I ran a temperature as high as 106°F and was hospitalized for several weeks. At that time I was on L-dopa but do not know how the medication was handled.

The illness or the medication seemed to influence food intake and weight control. The first effect of L-dopa was an increased desire for sweets. I wasn't quite aware of it but I must have bought more candy, and I gained about 10 pounds during the first period. During the summer of 1978 I became aware that my food habits had changed, in a specific setting. I went to Switzerland with a friend, and we selected a good hotel on account of its indoor swimming pool (the use of which did not help my poor coordination) and an especially good dining room. I was surprised how little I ate of the excellent food, and several times the maître d' inquired whether something was wrong. I began to select foods with the definite intent to gain weight and ate "fattening" foods that formerly had been definitely "no-no." I had the feeling that the extra movements, like the tremor and the rigidity, made a caloric demand just as if they were real exercise.

In 1978 I began to feel that L-dopa and carbidopa were less effective. I developed hyperkinesis, with dramatic choreiform movements. I made a peculiar observation: my friends who had rarely if ever commented on the shaking reacted strongly against the hyperkinesis. My inner reaction was the opposite: I experienced the tremor and rigidity as rather disturbing but had little reaction to the more coarse hyperkinetic movements. The time span between effective doses, with decrease in tremor and rigidity and appearance of hyperkinetic movements, became shorter and shorter. Dr. Cooper suggested that I take the carbidopa in smaller doses, every 2 h. I attempted this but found "every ten minutes, two hours are up."

I became more selective about traveling and invitations. However, I did keep it up and did not feel that traveling was too strenuous until the summer of 1981. Earlier that year I had received several invitations, with the host providing an escort. I found that I needed little extra help to travel on a plane; the hostesses are very helpful. The difficulty in traveling was the change in time zones and orienting myself in a hotel or conference halls.

It was in summer 1981 that I contemplated for the first time what it would mean to become an invalid. I reacted in what I now feel was an exaggerated way. I had accepted three invitations in Canada and Dallas, practically home territory, but I couldn't face the difficulties. When I mentioned this, that I had canceled engagements, Dr. Cooper felt the time had come for me to be tested on a new medication. He referred me to another neurologist who is in charge of the program to test a new drug.

My reaction to the new medication was rather dramatic. To supervise the drug action hospitalization for about 10 days was necessary. As far as I know, it didn't unfavorably affect my circulation, blood pressure, digestion, or other functions. But it did have a decided influence on my sleeping, memory, and style of thinking; also on my appetite. Except for a very brief period when I took bromocriptine my sleep had been excellent, and all Parkinson's symptoms stopped during the night. With the new medication I suddenly found myself stiff and somewhat rigid in bed, I could not straighten out my legs, and I felt generally too tense to sleep. This reaction continued after my discharge from the hospital.

The dosage of the new drug was gradually increased. I remember the month of December and early January as a time of excessive fatigue and memory difficulties. The arrangement had been that I saw the neurologist every 2 weeks, returned the bottles with the unused medication, and received new capsules. I expected that the dosage of active medication would be different in various samples. Early in January I felt that my old symptoms had come back, so I assumed that this had been the week during which I received placebos, capsules without the active drug. I had been wrong in my assumption: it was the following week that I received empty capsules.

I was shocked by the extent of the symptoms; everything I had experienced thus far in mild form suddenly became very big. The muscle rigidity was so strong that it disturbed my sleep and also walking; the tremor was so intense that I could not write or handle papers. Everything would be flying around. The symptoms were so severe that I asked for an earlier return appointment, and the neurologist saw me within 2 days. I asked him whether the capsules had been without medication, and he confirmed that this was the case.

At that time I considered this the most difficult week since I had become acquainted with parkinsonism; the regular use of medication had camouflaged the progress of the illness. I turned for a description of Parkinson's illness to a text from my medical school years, a time that there was no effective medication, and this gave me a frightening picture of its potential severity.

I had lost some weight while hospitalized, and I attributed it to the quality of hospital food. But on coming home I didn't like the food I provided either, specifically I didn't touch ice cream. During that period I became alarmed about losing my appetite, because nothing sounds more dreadful to me than not to enjoy food. I had a double reaction: the first one was to "spoil" myself, tempt myself with special dishes. I did it by looking into my deep freeze and cabinets for special foods. I found three squabs, which I like very much and which made attractive meals. I also located special hors d'oeuvres like caviar and escargot and made it a habit to have some every evening as my "appetizer" until the dozen or so jars were gone. I was amused about the motivation: I had saved the goodies for special occasions and was afraid that I might lose my interest in them. In a way, it worked; within the 2 weeks or so that it took me to consume my special foods my interest had been rearoused, and I ate the ordinary food again. As a matter of fact, I ate sufficient amounts to regain some of the lost weight.

But I find that my food habits are definitely changed, partly as a decision to simplify housekeeping but mainly because I have become finicky with my appetite. My shopping list has become smaller and smaller, more items going on the "I don't care" list. Fortunately, my likes apply to enough foods so that I can maintain good nutrition. I am amused by the definiteness with which I refuse to eat foods that I used to like but are now on my "no longer interested" list. During the last 6 to 8 months I have started something I had never done before, namely, skipping meals. I am slightly bewildered that I don't have more hunger. I find that I am more alert in the afternoon when I have lunch, but it doesn't bother me in the least to skip it.

I was returned to active medication and some of the most severe symptoms disappeared. I forgot the exact reason why, but ethopropazine was added, I assume to help control the shaking. It was during the later weeks of January that the most dramatic mental difficulties became manifest. During December and the early part of January I had been excessively sleepy and forgetful. I canceled practically all invitations during the Christmas season, and I left early or fell asleep at the parties I did attend. The fatigue was so great that I fell asleep when reading, and the forgetfulness was so severe that I repeated myself over and over when dictating letters.

By late January I was terribly alarmed because I was not thinking straight. I had reported the difficulties with memory and the peculiar thinking, but I couldn't give examples because I did not recall what had gone on. The first observation was that I made misstatements while dictating notes on patients. I threw in a number of things that had not happened or did not relate to the particular patient, like speaking of her leaving the hospital against advice, whereas the patient had not been hospitalized at all.

The worst confusion occurred during the last week in January, when I was on increasing doses of the experimental drug but also took ethopropazine. On the whole, I had the feeling that the ethopropazine was responsible for the unclear thinking, but the most dramatic episode occured when the experimental drug dosage was raised. On the day that I first took this larger dose I felt fine during the morning, maybe better than usual because I had more adequate amounts of the medication. I took the second dose of 1 mg before lunch, which I had with a friend who later told me her observations. After lunch I became aware that something was drastically wrong. I walked as if I were drunk, and I couldn't concentrate on any particular thoughts. I recorded a consultation scheduled for that afternoon, and the tape was later transcribed. There was one thread of thought that was logical and direct, and it pursued the problems that needed clarification in the same way that I ordinarily do. But there were interfering thoughts of which I was aware, and I made an effort not to say them out loud. "Looseness of association" would be a good description. There were several episodes in which the patient mentioned something to which I responded appropriately at first but then introduced questions or statements that were confusing.

I had two more appointments that afternoon, with patients who knew about the parkinsonism and the new medication. These sessions went fairly well, even though I made a number of misstatements. One of these patients had a family member suffering from Parkinsonism and was actively interested in my reaction. About 20 min after we had discussed by predicament I suddenly was quite "sober" and from then on did not go off the track again. If anything, I was mentally more active than usual, alert, quite productive, and interested in a wide range of things. I felt at that time that "losing my mind" was a remarkable experience, and I liked talking about it, whereas some of my friends felt embarrassed about the openness with which I handled it.

Eventually, I became adjusted to the new medication, after the ethopropazine had been stopped. I had decidedly less tremor, and the hyperkinesis stopped completely. The difficulty was and still lies in the unevenness of control. I felt well enough to accept an invitation to give an out-of-town lecture and stay as visiting professor in April. Three days after my return I noticed new symptoms with tremor in both legs, so that I could scarcely walk, sometimes being really "frozen" to the spot. This diminished after 2 or 3 days but then came back full force in June and July.

I had been scheduled for a cataract operation early in June, and this operation went very well. But I had complicated it by falling and breaking my left arm 3 days earlier. Everything was well controlled during the hospitalization, but within the next few weeks I experienced something for which I was completely unprepared, severe motor inhibition accompanied by excruciating pain in the left leg. The pain abated after 2 weeks when the dosage of carbidopa/L-dopa was changed. But even after relief from the pain my ability to walk was greatly impaired. For several weeks I was unable to leave my apartment but shuffled around as well as I could and kept on working.

By early September the walking difficulties were severe, and my sense of well-being was affected, so I was rehospitalized for evaluation and readjustment of the medication. Unfortunately, there was little change, even with a new medication schedule. I also underwent a medical checkup for some dyspnea that appeared when I tried to walk, but no measurable abnormality was found. I was discharged on condition of having a constant companion to protect me against falling, It would make for interesting reading to describe the various misadventures with a whole series of nurses and sitters. I managed better with members of my own family. But the question of a live-in protector is still unsettled.

SUMMARY

My reaction to parkinsonism for the first 8 or 9 years amounted practically to a denial of illness, not facing the fact that I was suffering from a serious chronic illness. My attitude toward the medications was not only accepting but I attributed nearly magical powers to them. I am still surprised that I reacted to the decreasing range of activities with so little depression, self-pity, or feeling excluded.

My reaction to the illness underwent a dramatic change during the last few months, when I suffered the severe inability to walk and needed help for the simplest activities. I experienced this inability as completely crippling, and I resented the personal help I needed. A week after I had been discharged from the hospital (with a companion) I suffered an acute febrile episode with signs of delirium. In retrospect it seems to have been a toxic reaction to the various medications, without an infection. The symptoms disappeared in a dramatic way. On a much smaller dosage I have practically no symptoms at all except hyperkinetic reaction to the carbidopa/L-dopa. The relief has persisted until now (time of writing, end of September 1982).

I am not sure whether I would have managed the illness differently if I had not protected myself by denial. I do not know whether it would have been of help if my physicians had been more outspoken and in a way prepared me for the difficult periods. I am aware of and familiar with the double bind of being realistic versus being optimistic. If I were asked whether I would participate again in an experimental drug study, I am sure my first answer would be an outspoken no. But this would be balanced by the question of what the progress of the illness would have been without it. In a peculiar way this illness has left me more trusting and hopeful, with greater reliance on finding help not only from physicians, whose dedication I gratefully acknowledge, but also from many friends and unknown bystanders.

On December 14, 1984, Dr. Hilde Bruch died. The following addendum to her chapter was written on November 7, 1984. "Since the paper was given . . . I became increasingly invalid (ed) and needed more and more continuous care. (Over the next year) I became increasingly fatigued and unstable. . . . Constipation became a conspicuous symptom and when I finally had this specifically examined it turned out to be the effect of a malignancy which had invaded the whole pelvic region. I have since learned that a combination of this order is rare, but when it occurs, it takes the form of increasing the severity of Parkinsonism. . . . The main point is still true, that I had an unusually optimistic attitude during the first years of the illness, so much so that I overlooked the development of a serious other illness."

REFERENCES

Dorros, S. (1981). *Parkinson's: A patient's view.* Washington, DC: Seven
    Locks Press.
Duvoisin, R. C. (1978). *Parkinson's disease: A guide for patient and family.*
    New York: Raven Press.

Chapter 11

EMOTIONAL PROBLEMS IN THE MANAGEMENT OF CANCER

Avery D. Weisman

THE CANCER PLIGHT AND PSYCHOSOCIAL EFFECTIVENESS

The plight of the cancer patient is unique among chronic diseases. Although other diseases may carry an even worse prognosis, cancer carries a significance that is both real and symbolic. For most people, and for a surprising number of physicians and health professionals, cancer symbolizes almost everything that is deadly, destructive, and inexorable. Consequently, the diagnosis of cancer the disease is apt to be confused with cancer the metaphor; as a result patients tend to become very apprehensive, and doctors may consider all treatment as merely temporizing. In our efforts to "win the war against cancer" these cultural biases are frequently overlooked.

I do not emphasize this somber side of cancer in order to discourage positive efforts to educate and manage effectively. On the contrary, the peculiarly frightening implications of cancer require special attention to the emotional and psychosocial overload. To treat the tumor without also heeding the personal plight of the patient is inadequate.

Coping with cancer entails more than surgery, chemotherapy, and radiation (Ahmed, 1981). Whether or not a trained professional is involved, there are few cancer patients who do not have psychosocial problems to contend with. This fact is well known to oncology nurses and social workers. Cancer treatment cannot be given with confidence unless possible sources of distress are recognized. To be thorough, we also ought to know more about the social unit of which the patient is a part.

There are four principal parts to consider in evaluating the cancer plight: (1) site, (2) situation, (3) social supports, and (4) self, or personality of the patient. For completeness we should include the care givers and the significant others, but their problems are beyond the scope of this presentation.

Site

The actual site of a cancer may be more threatening to a patient than its medical prognosis and treatability. The same can be said about disability imposed by treatment and the relation of site and treatment to later psychosocial interactions.

More specifically, the question is to what extent emotional distress is aggravated by visibility, disability, and social implications? For example, removal of a malignant melanoma from the face will literally change a patient's self-image as well as his or her inferences about what other people think. This is more than a cosmetic factor, because a similar situation arises with patients who have had different kinds of bowel surgery, with and without a colostomy. Emotional problems of mastectomy patients are well known, but similar disfigurement occurs with other cancers too.

Situation

Only in experimental animals does a tumor exist independently of the psychosocial situation. There is even doubt if this is true of experimental tumors. We can be reasonably sure that the cancer situation is affected by threats to job, finances, marriage, parenting, and many other aspects of what it takes to get along, thrive, and fulfill conventional roles. Some patients adapt and get along without significant complications, whereas others are practically devastated. Most situations are in between in severity, just as most patients are vulnerable to a degree. The important point, I believe, is that the diagnosis and treatment of cancer are likely to infringe on many important attitudes and activities, and these impediments are seldom investigated by personnel who are primarily engaged in treating tumors.

Social Supports

Although we do not have matched controls to study the effect of social support on survival, recovery, and relapse after cancer treatment, we do know that intervention by health professionals does make a significant difference in how readily and persistently patients adapt themselves. Since the practice of psychosocial intervention varies greatly, it is plausible that the positive benefit of heeding psychosocial issues in patients may be due to increasing social supports. Few patients are able to get along by themselves without help during convalescence. Material and social assistance is required, if only to the extent that someone significant cares. Sick patients in general are more vulnerable, their quality of life is impaired, morale is damaged, and they need the supportive presence or availability of outside resources to keep from feeling helpless.

Self

The factor of personality hardly needs emphasis, since people vary in capacity to deal with problems and to muster adequate coping efforts. Nevertheless, to be diagnosed as having cancer is as serious and as significant an occasion for self-appraisal as any moment that is likely to happen. If we, as clinicians, cannot appreciate the impact of the fact of cancer, then we cannot deal with its consequences. The personality trait of optimism versus pessimism is likely to be a decisive predictive point for anticipating distress later in the course. As a rule, how well a person will cope with cancer and its treatment is partially reflected in how that individual coped with previous problems, less life-threatening.

I have found the phrase *psychosocial effectiveness* to be more useful than generalities about adaptation, adjustment, or even acclimatization. It is the effectiveness of how we manage and cope that is important because the process undergoes constant change, and seldom reaches a point of equilibrium when no activity is noted. Psychological entropy does not exist, except postmortem. Psychosocial effectiveness demands frequent evaluation because it involves specific tasks and problems. To learn about a problem is a necessary attribute of considering various strategies for solving it. As a doctor, I may teach you, but you instruct yourself.

Combining attention to site, situation, social supports, and self permits a more comprehensive evaluation of distress throughout the course of cancer.

COMMON EMOTIONAL PROBLEMS IN CANCER

Because the human condition is what it is, immersed in ambiguity, ambivalence, anxiety, and apprehension, not every emotional or psychosocial difficulty should or could be attributed to cancer, even with a very generous definition. Expectable emotional problems are really instances of psychosocial ineffectiveness in coping, since coping and distress have an inverse relationship. A pertinent emotional problem, therefore, is a distressing situation that compromises efforts to cope by oneself and is likely to impede cancer treatment, management, or sustained periods of recovery.

There is much overlapping between problems not related to cancer and those that impede cancer care. Some problems are immediately recognized; others are noted to be a potential threat, whereas still other problems are diagnosed only in retrospect. For example, we are not sure which marriages are threatened by a child's leukemia or other malignancy. We do have evidence of the deleterious effect of childhood cancer on a shaky parental marriage. Marital incompatibility may be increased by another emotional burden, such as a child's cancer. But the marital problems probably preceded the illness and might have resulted in the parents' closing ranks when their child became ill. Similar considerations apply to any cancer-related situation that has consequences for psychosocial changes.

Potential obstacles to proper management of cancer are found largely in personal concerns about *diagnosis, treatment, prognosis, persistent symptoms,* and *nonmedical complications* and *consequences.* We have no clear evidence that I know about that prognosis is adversely affected or promoted by emotional distress, although there are hints in both directions. It is sufficient to note, however, that those who cope better have a better quality of life and undergo treatment with less distress. Our emphasis should be on vulnerable occasions related to cancer in which management can be impaired or the patient adversely affected.

Here are ten such problem areas:

1. Impact of diagnosis
2. Effects of primary treatment
3. Preoccupation with symptoms, potential complications, discontinuous, or unreliable health care
4. Expectations for good or ill; optimism or pessimism; worries, woes, and discontents
5. Disruption or dissolution of social supports and other interpersonal changes
6. Isolation, abandonment, and repudiation of and by significant others
7. Personal devaluation on basis of job, responsibilities, finances, and self-appraisal
8. Encroachment on self-autonomy
9. Dysphoria, disposition, and deviant behavior
10. Existential concerns, demoralization, despair

Impact of Diagnosis

Patients have a right to know their diagnosis, not simply for legal purposes but because secrecy is bad practice. Few patients can be fooled for very long; the question is not whether to tell but how to tell effectively, honestly, and tactfully. Physicians generally fear this duty, because it affects their compassion and later on their sense of competence.

Understandably, some patients become distraught, but the

acute distress subsides within a day or two. Distress among significant others will last longer, but with help and support it can be redirected to supporting the patient. Not infrequently, however, the patient comes to support the family later on. Care givers should not be surprised that one session offering information may not be enough. Information does not get through. Patients may deny, show middle-knowledge, or do flip-flops about their motivation to continue treatment.

Although the existential plight of life-threatening information typically occurs after the diagnosis and for a short period into convalescence, some patients wholly expect and anticipate cancer by the time they first present themselves. The prediagnostic period has to do with delay, anticipation, and expectation for good or ill.

Effects of Primary Treatment

Every form of treatment has built-in potential for impediment. Some are self-evident, such as mastectomy or colostomy; others are less tangible and easily confused with psychological issues, such as weariness, depression, and vague pains associated with radiation.

Side effects of treatment can be predicted to some extent, but primary emotional effects of treatment are more personal and less related to the modality itself. The central point is that patients may blame themselves and be afraid of being blamed further by care givers for any idiosyncratic response.

Preoccupation with Symptoms, Potential Complications, and Discontinuous, or Unreliable Health Care

Patients are afraid of bothering doctors with complaints, even in this day of emancipation and second opinions. But it is even more surprising to learn how often doctors are fooled into thinking patients have no complaints or problems because they do not hear them. On one hand, hypochondriasis is diagnosed more frequently than is justified. On the other hand, existential qualms about survival at all are diagnosed less often. In between are patients and families worried about not being able to maintain communication and deserving the attention of their physician. For example, a group of widows was asked what advice they would give to someone else just starting on the course they had completed with their husbands. The answer, almost unanimously, was that they would insist on getting more information from the doctor and, in general, would find a physician who was more accessible and available. None asked for a miraculous cure; all wanted someone who would care over the long run. It is for the long run as well as for management of potential complications and persistent consequences that the visiting nurses fit in so admirably.

Expectations for Good or Ill; Optimism or Pessimism; Worries, Woes, and Discontents

It is no secret that optimists generally cope better with cancer, regardless of the ultimate outcome. They are more resourceful and use resources better than those who are habitual pessimists. It is one thing to be duly skeptical about extravagant promises of total recovery but quite another to despair of the treatment that is available and to feel that one is merely borrowing time against the inevitable. Furthermore, pessimists do not even have the consolation of their own conviction. They tend to have more woes and worries and have higher average distress. Optimists and pessimists, we believe, have intermittent bouts of despondency of the same frequency and intensity.

Disruption or Dissolution of Social Supports, and Other Interpersonal Changes

Although we rarely hear about bias, prejudice, and discrimination against cancer patients at work or in social situations, it exists. Some patients are more perceptive of these attitudes than others. In the English language there is no satisfactory term for a close acquaintance who is neither a fellow-worker nor a friend. Consequently, patients may expect more from so-called friends than is justified. Friends may quickly disappear on one pretext or another, leaving support and necessary householding tasks to somewhat less reluctant family members. The old-fashioned extended family about whom so much romantic nonsense is written is seldom found in an urban culture. Patients must then, more realistically, find social supports among professional care givers or volunteers who have taken up the cause.

Isolation, Abandonment, and Repudiation of and by Significant Others

Some patients simply cannot hold up their end of a relationship, or they insist on solitude. Much of this may be attributed to loss of personal self-esteem as well as to resentment about enforced inactivity. Repudiation of and by significant others refers to close friends and family. It is a self-perpetuating, mutually destructive cycle of request and reluctance, blame and shame, silence and guilt, bitterness and inappropriate behavior.

Personal Devaluation on Basis of Job, Responsibilities, Finances, and Self-Appraisal

These problems constitute a conglomerate of reasons why some cancer patients think poorly of themselves and are ashamed to admit it. To be workless, in our society, is to be practically worthless, even through no personal fault. The idea is that we are dispensable, almost throwaways. The sick role is essentially nonproductive; mothers find it difficult to function as before, and fathers fail to provide for their families. Devaluation of self is disability of the spirit and may be as incapacitating as actual invalidism. If patients begin to feel like just another case, it is understandable when they talk of little besides their symptoms, since that is all that makes them interesting. One of the strongest elements in maintaining an appropriate quality of life is an effort to bring about continuity between this cancer phase and earlier periods of health.

Encroachment on Self-Autonomy

Autonomy means the ability to think out alternatives and to act according to one's best interests. With certain cancer situations dependence, if not semi-invalidism, is the rule. Soon patients feel unable to speak up for themselves and then to have no right to want more than they are given. Self-reliance is a measure of autonomy; even in families where devotion and dedication are the reigning concerns, exhaustion occurs, patients know it, and then autonomy becomes compromised.

Dysphoria, Disposition, and Deviant Behavior

There are no problems without a degree of dysphoria, i.e., a concomitant unpleasant emotion. In practical terms, although we may expect that a certain situation will cause a problem, if a patient reports no distress or fails to show an equivalent aberration, we cannot insist on our version. Conversely, when a patient complains about distress, such as in chronic pain, and we as physicians are at a loss to find a reason or problem to account for the pain, our tendency is tacitly to blame the victim. To recognize dysphoria is only to find a direction, not to make a diagnosis.

Most dysphorias have a corresponding disposition or type of behavior that is designed to do away with the painful emotion. For example, someone who is afraid of drug addiction will refuse to fill prescriptions, lie about his misbehavior, or split the dose without telling anyone.

The problem of dysphoria is especially relevant these days, when medications are available. The diagnosis of "depression" is made more often, instead of the other way around, as it was when depression was considered somewhat socially unrespectable, and there were practically no medications for it.

I maintain that because the diagnosis is being made more often, the characteristics of depression have become more poorly defined. DSM-III has given us only the features of relatively severe depression, not the depressions of everyday life. Unipolar depression differs from grief, sadness, morose feelings, or discontent associated with sluggishness, slowed-down sexual responses, poor appetite, and neuromuscular fatigue. The depression encountered in and by cancer patients is seldom that of unipolar depression; despair is more low-keyed than in presuicidal patients. Middle age counts many cancer patients, and so-called depression of middle years may be aggravated by the diagnosis, treatment, and existential uncertainty of cancer.

It is relatively easy to recognize the dysphoria of unspoken anger, less easy to know about silent depression, and very difficult to get a nonspecific anxiety. I prefer to diagnose *dysphoric mood disturbance* rather than prematurely pinning a patient's feeling down to anxiety or depression. Moreover, since we are concerned about emotional problems, it is less important to categorize the emotion itself than to associate dysphoria with disposition to behave in certain tension-relieving ways. Getting a fix on the time, place, and situation may disclose the basic problems.

Existential Concerns, Demoralization, Despair

A cancer patient who is not moved to examine and question his or her own existence, values, and life trajectory is either unusually obtuse or simply misleading the interviewer. As I have indicated, cancer is a metaphor for the transience of life and the ever-presence of death in most of what we do. But beyond the existential jolt of cancer diagnosis, patients come to terms with uncertainty, even forgetting about it, just like ordinary people. Nevertheless, existential concerns face mankind, and cancer patients, at every turn of illness and treatment. Naturally, few patients present themselves in quite this way. However, when asked about how they think of themselves and their situation, many respond with statements such as "I wish I'd gone to church more often," or as one patient put it, "When I get to heaven, I have a bone to pick with God!" Still others say, "I don't mind for myself, but my children are just too young to bear up under all this. What will happen to them, after I'm gone?"

Demoralization is, in my opinion, the basic distinction between a patient who can cope reasonably well and one who is on the edge of despair. When demoralization sets in, patients have lost confidence that they can undertake any measure on their own behalf, or that anything at all can be done, regardless of the realistic facts. Destiny is doom.

PERIODS OF SIGNIFICANT VULNERABILITY

With few exceptions, expectable problems can occur almost at any time. However, in actual practice problems tend to

bunch, pyramid, or snowball at expectable transitions. Therefore, knowing about the following transitions will alert care givers to the likelihood that inquiry into personal matters at such
moments may be rewarding and necessary.

1. On first becoming a cancer patient
2. During and shortly after primary treatment
3. While undergoing prolonged convalescence and its
   consequences
4. While trying to resume regular life and ordinary rou-
   tines
5. In cases of extended uncertainty and limbo
6. At times of surprise or unsurprise related to relapse
   and recurrence
7. Receiving minimal benefit while being treated for
   metastasis
8. Posttherapeutic decline; preterminal sickness unto
   death

There is an advantage in lengthening the list of high-risk
transition points. Otherwise, clinicians might overlook vulnerable periods, and assume that all is well, or that because distress
is expectable, it needs no further attention.

Generally speaking, patients seem to have their own level
of vulnerability, i.e., disposition to be distressed, regardless of
extrinsic difficulties. That is, there are patients who typically
show higher distress than others, and when they do, levels of
distress are always higher, though apt to vary, depending on the
problem or transition point. Most patients are comparatively
quiescent during symptom-free remissions. But patients with
higher average distress will be still more distressed during remissions than those who are habitually less distressed.

The peak periods for distress in either group are at times
of diagnosis and recurrence. The posttherapeutic period might
be expected to be devastating. Although some patients, having
denied and disbelieved, finally are confronted with unbeliev-
able facts, the chronic deniers continue to deny. Most scales that
measure distress depend on truthfulness, and those who deny
maintain their posture that hardly anything is wrong. I cannot

claim, however, that deniers are generally less distressed, because they often have many somatic difficulties that replace emotional anguish.

An important implication of these findings is the likelihood that if a patient copes well at the onset of cancer, he or she will cope satisfactorily and with less distress throughout its course. We have noted that with patients in the preterminal period, distress is far less than anticipated by healthy people who can only imagine what this phase is like.

CONCEPT OF VULNERABILITY

I have already suggested that separation of painful or dysphoric affect into anxiety, anger, and depression is far too simple. The range of emotion is too wide and individualized to be covered adequately in these terms. Furthermore, diagnostic criteria for emotional disturbance are not agreed on, and most clinicians have their private standards that rating scales only confirm.

Consider, for instance, patients who show a variety of emotions, all of which might qualify as dysphoria: grief, loneliness, jealousy, frustration, bewilderment, guilt, worry, shame, self-pity, and so on. Combine these with a variety of coping strategies and defenses. The desirability of a more accurate assessment of emotion is self-evident. In that way only can specific distress signals be interpreted. Recall too that dysphoria is a sign of distress related to lack of coping effectiveness and therefore may foreshadow an impediment to cancer management.

The most sensitive and simplest assessment of how well or poorly a cancer patient copes is merely asking about *morale*. Like most other important concepts, definition is imprecise, but most people know what they mean and feel. In my opinion, good morale consists of competent coping, a sense of confidence, and a belief that, all things considered, we are at our best. Fear of failure, giving up completely, falling into a state of nothingness, and despairing of any positive change are signs of *demoralization*, the ultimate dysphoria. Good morale can be acknowledged readily and easily differentiated from another form of vulnerability that I call *existential denial*, where there is much self-congratulatory positive thinking as well as repudiation of even normal difficulties.

I propose that clinicians pay attention not only to what patients say or report about themselves but to what patients are observed to do, say, or report when the clinician is not around. Behavior at home may be more revealing than behavior in the doctor's office or the hospital, when roles are quite different. Some coping strategies are active; others, passive. Which tendency is selected depends on habit, custom, availability, approval, circumstances, and of course, a patient's assessment of what a problem calls for.

DISTRESS AMONG CARE GIVERS

In recent months, not more than a year or two, references to "burnout" among care givers seem to have increased or at least come out of the closet. It is difficult to recall discussion of this topic in earlier times, when professionalism seemed to require a more "scientific" attitude of detachment. Now, with more emphasis on holistic care, care givers feel freer to examine their own feelings and contributions and to be open about it. I encourage this trend, because in my opinion there are few reactions in patients that cannot also occur among care givers. Consequently, emotional problems among care givers may inadvertently impose obstacles and impediments in the management of cancer too. I would define a more general syndrome, less conspicuous than burnout, that I call "care giver's plight": a syndrome caused by promises gone awry, efforts gone unrecognized, professional activities that fall short, producing distress, demoralization, a sense of defeat, incompetence, and hopelessness (Weisman, 1981).

Distress signals include such indicators as aversion to patients; abhorrence of work; phony optimism about prognosis; denial of fallibility; sudden pangs, tears, and wipeouts; unnatural, even magical expectations of sudden reverses, and so on.

STRATEGIC GUIDELINES FOR PSYCHOSOCIAL MANAGEMENT

I wish it were possible to set down a set of guidelines that every clinician could practice and become adept at. I can only suggest a few large principles, which I have detailed in another place (Weisman, 1979): collaboration with the patient; confrontation and recognition of salient problems to be coped with; co-operating in affording tactical relief and control; and modulating emotional extremes.

What are the *aims in management* of cancer patients that if achieved signify coping well enough to avoid major emotional obstacles?

1. Available and accessible health care, including management of symptoms and support by and of others
2. Participation in major decisions, or at least enough information to yield decision to trusted significant other
3. Reduction of distress, so that emotions are kept within bounds that do not warp judgment
4. Open information and ample communication about various procedures and events related to management
5. Preservation as much as possible of positive elements and satisfactions stemming from healthier days
6. Coordinating treatment goals with psychosocial management, so that surprise and shock are minimized
7. Affording opportunities and resources for correcting nonmedical, psychosocial difficulties

SUMMARY

1. Emotional problems in management of cancer are determined by whatever has the potential of impeding management, convalescence, recovery, or the ability to cope.
2. Emotional distress is manifested by different signals;

depression is by no means the only or even the most important dysphoric affect.

3. Demoralization is the major indicator of emotional problems. The maintenance of morale is the major indicator of coping capacity.

4. Painful emotions such as conspicuous anger, depression, and anxiety signify only extreme versions of vulnerability. They provide a direction for further investigation and assessment and are not diagnoses in themselves.

5. Care givers need to heed their own emotional responses, because objectivity and efficiency vary with emotions. How a care giver feels is apt to influence assessment of how patients feel.

6. Truth is desirable, but tactful intervention, combining compassion with candor, is an indispensable guideline.

7. Compassion with candor does not compromise good treatment, nor does it exclude thorough evaluation.

REFERENCES

Ahmed, P. (1981). *Living and dying with cancer*. New York: Elsevier–North Holland.

Weisman, A. D. (1979). *Coping with cancer*. New York: McGraw-Hill.

Weisman, A. D. (1981). Understanding the cancer patient: The syndrome of caregiver's plight. *Psychiatry, 44,* 161–168.

Chapter 12

PSYCHOLOGICAL ADJUSTMENT TO PHYSICAL TRAUMA AND DISABILITY

David W. Krueger

SIGNIFICANCE OF TRAUMA OR DEFECT

The psychological significance and impact of physical trauma and defect depends on some combination of the following elements (Castelnuovo-Tedesco, 1981):

1. Time of acquisition (especially vis-á-vis place in the life cycle)
2. Size and location of defect
3. Effect on general health
4. Size of lesion
5. Internal/external; visible/nonvisible
6. Permanent/temporary/capable of physical restitution
7. Predictable/unpredictable
8. Loss/addition of body parts
9. Nature of the trauma
10. Whether the trauma can be consciously remembered
11. Preexisting personality/psychopathology of the individual
12. Preceding losses

The issues of acquired loss and trauma are not present if the defect is congenital or perinatal. Even though loss itself is not an issue, the defect is still woven intricately into a self-image. It may become a hook onto which various difficulties and failures are hung.

There is always an element of trauma, both physically and emotionally, in acquired injuries. Physical losses such as sensation, mobility, sexual functioning, cognitive facility, and bowel and bladder control are always concurrent in some degree with emotional losses of status, job functioning, present as well as future goals, and diminished self-esteem.

If the physical defect is acquired through trauma or disease process, it is important to know what phase of psychological development it interferes with and whether there have been significant losses that preceded it. A greater immunity from significant emotional disturbance due to a physical loss is granted with greater emotional stability, age, developmental maturity, and no significant unresolved preceding losses, physically or emotionally.

STAGES OF PSYCHOLOGICAL ADJUSTMENT

One of the most significant variables that determines how traumatic the physical insult will be is the capacity of the insult either to provoke regression or to stimulate adaptive coping in the patient. This can be fully understood only in the context of a patient's own individual development, coupled with an assessment and understanding of the normal and expectable stages of adaptation the patient progressed through at the time of physical trauma and disability and following it. The five stages I will outline usually are all present in some form and degree in a healthy psychological adaptation to physical disability. Impediments to emotional rehabilitation usually manifest as difficulty in negotiating one of these stages or as the persistence of one stage obstructing further movement. The stages that will be discussed are (1) shock, (2) denial, (3) depressive reaction, (4) reaction against independence, and (5) adaptation (Krueger, 1982).

Shock

The immediate reaction to a trauma is a sense of shock, a state of nonintegration of excessive overwhelming stimuli. One is unable to integrate or comprehend the magnitude or the severity of the event, not even its immediate consequences. This state of numbness is both emotional and physical. It may last for a period of moments or up to several days. Emergency care teams are frequently the only ones outside the immediate family to observe this part of the patient's experience.

Denial

When confronted with trauma, patients use existing inner models to interpret the new events (Horowitz & Kaltreider, 1977). Those models that have been developed in the past must be used to interpret the present. When loss occurs, new information confronts an existing model, and the result is an acute disequilibrium. The response to this transition may initially be shock, followed by a denial of the recognition coupled with numbing of emotions. Denial allows the individual to act as if nothing has changed and as if no loss had occurred. The intrusion of reality and denial or avoidance of reality is not sudden, total, or all-or-nothing. Instead it tends to oscillate in a gradually emerging pattern that is highly individual (Khann & Masund, 1963). These intrusive experiences and alternating denial or avoidance are the essential elements of posttraumatic disorders (Horowitz & Kaltreider, 1977).

The universal initial reaction is denial. This position is initially most useful, because it is beyond the capacity of any individual to accept such a sudden and drastic change in his/her body image and self-concept.

During this phase of response there is as yet no depression. Depression does not exist because there is no conscious acknowledgment of the permanence or severity of the loss; denial has insured that. Depression, the response to the recognition of loss, is delayed until the patient actually perceives the extent of this dilemma and emotionally recognizes that irreparable loss has occurred.

Although the process of denial is adaptive and protective

to insure against being overwhelmed initially, the denial should gradually soften to allow the patient to comprehend and integrate his/her loss and recognize its consequences. Only when denial is extended and becomes maladaptive (interferes with rehabilitative efforts) should intervention be effected.

Depressive Reaction

Denial gradually gives way to a fuller recognition and comprehension of the severity and extent of the loss or illness. At this point grief and depression emerge. The denial to this point has not been of the *reality* of the event but of its *significance, seriousness,* and *permanence.* The patient may have felt that the lost limb or function is still intact although perhaps not currently functioning fully. Dreams and daydreams have served as a reparative fantasy in which one is functioning wholly and intactly. Vigorous rehabilitative efforts often abruptly confront the patient with the now undeniable evidence of an irreversible loss.

Depression is present at this point of the recognition of loss. It is a normal response and is to be expected as a reaction to a severe illness or loss of body part or function. If it does not occur, even transiently, an alarm should sound, because its absence indicates that the reality of the loss has not been emotionally recognized. Another aspect of depression is a reaction to an awareness of helplessness in maintaining self-esteem. If the lost part or function is intimately related to self-esteem, the patient may be unable to maintain a sense of self-esteem; depression will then ensue. It is important to assess how the patient maintained self-esteem prior to his/her injury and how the loss suffered has altered these efforts.

The emotional significance of the loss must be determined for each patient. A loss that interferes with cognitive processes is more devastating for the patient whose career, recreation, self-esteem, and defensive and coping mechanisms are predicated on intellectual functioning. The patient whose esteem, work, coping, interests, and life-styles are centered around physical activities will have a more marked reaction and greater difficulty in adjustment when a physical debilitation occurs.

Depression, anxiety, sadness, grief, and anger are to be expected as natural and appropriate. Some impairment of self-esteem also will occur, manifesting as a sense of helplessness, feeling oneself to be a burden to others, and feeling that one has nothing to offer others. Depressions caused by physical disability are more reality-based than depressive disorders based on neurotic mechanisms of guilt, unexpressed hostility, or narcissistic emptiness (Steiger, 1976). Adding to the sense of helplessness and depression is the sudden ineffectiveness of the patient's old behaviors in bringing about self-enhancing responses from others, not that he/she is disabled.

When one feels particularly helpless regarding a physical condition and unable to master even basic functions in one's body, the idea of suicide is often conceived as an alternative way to achieve a sense of mastery. At least one has control over one's life. Particularly for the patient who has little control over his/her life, body, or environment, this ultimate control over the continuation or cessation of his/her life has important psychological significance. The recognition by the treating person of this need and the acknowledgment of the purpose this serves from an adaptive standpoint can be extremely helpful—to put a patient's feelings and despair into words, such as "I can understand how you would want to have some control over your own life; at least for right now it seems as though there is little control over what is happening to you and even your own body."

Often the progress of the patient's emotional rehabilitation can be followed and indexed by the content of dreams, daydreams and phantom pain. Dreams that progressively recognize the current state of loss (e.g., paraplegia) indicate a more complete mourning process than dreams and daydreams that persist in representing the person in a pre-loss state, as if nothing had happened. The recognition of grief and confrontation of denial parallel the effectiveness of the mourning process and are concomitant with the depressive phase of reaction. Similarly, a traumatic episode that might be repeatedly experienced in daydreams as frightening and realistic may, as mourning proceeds, be detoxified and assimilated. Phantom pain that is persistent beyond the period when it is primarily physically based indicates the emotional need to perceive the limb as "still there" even if painfully so. With progressive recognition, mourning, and giving up what was and what might have been, a memory is created—a memory of the trauma, of one's previous potential, goals, and body image. These are mourned to allow the recognition of new potential goals and new perceptions of oneself. Through this mourning process depressive reactions are resolved.

Reaction against Independence

Some patients may react against autonomy, self-care, and leaving the hospital, consciously or unconsciously. This reaction against independence is particularly noteworthy in two groups of patients. One group includes late adolescents and young adults, for whom autonomy, separation, and independence are so new, untried, or recently achieved that any regression to a dependent posture is threatening. When this dependent posture is assumed in order to be a patient, it increases the difficulty of separation and autonomy from the hospital. For another group of patients, with long-standing latent or overt conflicts in relation to dependency versus independence, tipping the scales toward dependence in fulfilling the need for physical nursing care may make the withdrawal of fulfilling nursing care problematic.

Normal personality traits will be exaggerated at a time of stress, particularly at the time of an insult to one's bodily and emotional integrity. Any stress causes a heightened use of previously used defense mechanisms. The dependent patient will be more dependent; the conscientious, responsible patient will intensify his/her independence in an effort to compensate for the disability. Some traits are more adaptive for different phases of the patient role. For example, allowing oneself to be dependent and taken care of within limits and without marked protest works well during the initial phase, whereas being independent works better during rehabilitation efforts. Some defensive patterns work well during neither phase; for example, the borderline patient who has no consistent internal sense of self or goals adapts poorly during all phases of care. The particular ways in which grief is displayed also varies in accordance with the patient's personality.

Adaptation

A loss of body integrity or function evokes grief and mourning. There is mourning for the function, for the body image, for the satisfactions that the function gave that are now impossible. There is also grieving for the loss of future expectations that were based on the assumption of having that function. After the grief and mourning for these losses proceeds to the relinquishment of the hope for return, new roles and new expectations can be achieved; these are based on new potentials while acknowledging new limitations.

The predominant strategies of coping used by a patient can be maximized to help him/her in rehabilitation efforts (Stewart, 1978). Coping strategies and defense mechanisms are not exactly the same. Defense mechanisms are intrapsychic and operate unconsciously to avoid anxiety, depression, or psychic pain; they are formed initially in response to internal conflicts. Coping strategies operate consciously and involve the process of adapting reasonably and advantageously to the environment. Changes of great magnitude, especially those changes that defy solution with familiar patterns of behavior, are supreme tests of one's coping ability.

A working alliance with the patient who has experienced trauma is predicated on understanding both basic defense mechanisms and coping strategies. The coping strategies can be discovered by eliciting from the patient information about his customary way of handling other major stresses in his life. Like defense mechanisms, coping strategies tend to be consistent over time, and exacerbations of stress are met by an intensified use of coping strategies.

The list of coping strategies in Table 12-1 is an adaptation from Weisman (1974).

Among the major tasks of the treating professional is to determine the coping strategies utilized by a patient and to determine if the coping strategy will serve a positive purpose in rehabilitation. Those coping strategies that will augment and enhance rehabilitation and recovery would then be supported and further channeled into rehabilitation efforts, and maladaptive coping strategies would be redirected. For example, the pa-

Table 12-1. Predominant Coping Strategies

I. *Affective*
  A. Passivity, isolation of affect, and not worrying
  B. Denial and reversal of affect (laugh it off)
  C. Sharing feelings and reactions with others, with much talk about the adjustment
II. *Behavioral*
  A. Displacement and distraction with activities
  B. Confrontation with oneself and taking concerted action
  C. Acting out
  D. Repetition, using the same plans and activities as in previous stresses
  E. Avoidance and physical withdrawal from people and potential coping situations
III. *Cognitive*
  A. Rational-intellectual, seeking information and intellectual control
  B. Rationalization by redefinition: accepting and making a virtue out of the necessity
  C. Fatalism: stoic acceptance and preparation for the worst
  D. Projection and externalization, including blaming others
  E. Strict compliance with authority: doing as told
  F. Masochistic surrender: seeking blame, atonement, and self-sacrifice

tient who used displacement and immersion into activities could well utilize extremely active and early use of occupational and recreational therapy, with a full schedule of rehabilitative therapy on a more accelerated pace to meet his/her psychological as well as physical needs. Patients who use intellectualization as their primary coping mechanism should be allowed a reasonable amount of control and knowledge of diagnostic and treatment procedures. To such patients stress is a threat because it limits their ability to maintain control. An intellectually oriented patient may, for example, be allowed control by participation in treatment planning, coordination of treatment and rehabilitation efforts, and thorough explanations of his/her condition and procedures. Another patient, who would need to avoid and withdraw initially, may do much better with a far corner bed than with explanations.

DEPRESSIVE ILLNESS

What occurs when patients who experience a real external loss react with a major depressive *illness* rather than with grief and a transient depressive *reaction*? Some factors that predispose toward depressive illness in patients post-injury include a history of depressive illness, a family history of depression, and a predisposition toward depression. This predisposition includes such factors as a history of early parent loss and childhood trauma, overt or covert (Servoss & Krueger, 1984). The current traumatic loss may crystallize incomplete mourning of prior losses, including unresolved traumatic events or difficulty negotiating normal developmental tasks (Brown, 1961). In a previous study of a group of physical rehabilitation patients referred because of abnormal grief or overt depression following their injuries, we found a significantly high percentage (about 7 in every 10 patients) who had experienced the loss of a parent in childhood (Servoss & Krueger, 1984). A significant proportion of the remaining patients (3 of every 10) had experienced specific childhood traumas, especially physical abuse.

Trauma can be a sudden major event such as parent loss in childhood; long-standing situations accumulating frustrating tension, such as neglect or physical abuse; or major acute traumatic experiences. Trauma can be cumulative with overtly healthy functioning until overwhelmed by acute stress and crisis (Khann & Masund, 1963). A subsequent loss, such as physical illness or physical trauma, then interacts with earlier unresolved loss(es), with a reemergence of their associated emotions, such as helplessness and anger. The conflictual aspect of earlier trauma is the experience of passivity and helplessness, which lends a certain perspective to the perception of the current trauma. The emotional impact of the loss of the parent during the child's development, for example, may not be integrated and digested but is instead denied. This has a later impact on one's self-perceptions and object relationships (Krueger, 1983) and predisposes to the later development of clinical depression (Beck, Sethi, & Tuthill, 1963; Sethi, 1964).

Some patients experience such a narcissistic injury from their illness that they focus on their own predicament in an ever-increasing spiral of withdrawal of interest from others and the outside world, and finally invest interest only in themselves. For them, illness is seen as a loss of part of the self. "Their lives become self-centered and filled with a search for the self-state (health) which can never quite be regained" (Weiss, 1983). These patients may frequently shift from a denial of their illness to an exclusive preoccupation with their illness. What is lost is the ongoing fantasy of an ideal state of health, wholeness, invulnerability, and greatness. The secret ubiquitous fantasies of grandiosity, exhibitionism, immortality, omniscience, and omnipotence are closer to the surface in these people. In these people wishes for grandness alternate with a sense of inadequacy and poor self-esteem. Often there is an associated need to strive for perfection. A physical illness or trauma can be quite devastating to such persons, causing fluctuation between the poles of greatness on the one hand and inadequacy on the other, ultimately culminating in fixation on the pole of inadequacy, imperfection, and shame. This withdrawal is an attempt at self-repair, but the outcome may be only preoccupation with infinitely renewable fantasies of former function and with what might have been.

PRINCIPLES OF BRIEF THERAPY OF A TRAUMATIC EVENT

1. Begin at the level of the patient's immediate concerns.

For the liaison psychiatrist a review of the patient's physical condition with the consulting physician is necessary, as well as a review of the patient's chart. An initial working alliance is best established by introducing the psychiatrist, and by the psychiatrist introducing himself/herself, as a member of the medical team who is interested in helping with the emotional rehabilitation that is a crucial component of the medical-physical rehabilitation. The patient is not as inclined to feel singled out and "wacky" in having a consulting psychiatrist if this relationship to the medical team is established.

Discuss the currently perceived physical problem with the patient as a first order of business. This should begin with what is most on the surface, most conscious for the patient. This alleviates the patient's fear that his/her psychiatrist or therapist will delve deeply into emotional issues without first recognizing the most immediate and important problem to the patient.

2. Establish conditions that will help the patient process the traumatic event or the onset of illness.

The emotional aspects of the patient's experience must be woven into the account and the reliving of the experiences. Have the patient describe in detail the traumatic event. Affects reside in details. In a supportive manner this detail can be expanded to include emotional details such as reactions, feelings, ways of thinking, and ways of behaving. Elicit an account of the progression of events and experiences of the illness from onset to the present. Associations to the event and catharsis are essential.

3. Listen from the inside.

Empathic listening means an understanding of more than just the emotions of the patient. It means understanding of the entire psychological state, including a patient's perceptions, way of thinking, causal explanations, sense of self—his/her whole experiential state. Empathy does not mean being sympathetic, consoling, or commiserating. Empathy describes *a way of listening*—a particular vantage point of listening *from the inside*. One physician, Ralph Greenson (1967), describes how he uses it in the clinical situation:

> I change the way I am listening. . . . I shift from listening from the outside to listening from the inside. I have to let a part of me become the patient and I have to go through his experiences as if I were the patient and to introspect what is going on in me as they occur. . . . I let myself experience his associations, and his affects as he seems to have gone through them. . . . I go back over the patient's utter-

ances and transfer his words into pictures and feelings in accordance with his personality. I let myself associate to these pictures with his life experiences, his memories, his fantasies. . . . I have built up a working model of the patient. . . that I shift into the foreground as I try to capture what he was experiencing. (p. 367)

4. Assist the patient to work through, to accept the physical and emotional reality of loss—of what was, of what might have been, of what is now, and of what can be.

This work allows the past to be committed to memory rather than continuing as a painful, active, impeding, alive dynamic process. Energies can then be utilized to achieve full current and future potential, rather than to fixate on past potential.

5. Provide temporary medication as a component of this treatment if the symptoms are overwhelming or disruptive, or to assist the patient in dosing his/her feelings.

6. Termination is an integral component of the therapeutic work.

Termination is the end in mind from the beginning. Consolidation of previous work, implications and recommendations for the future are discussed. The therapist's ongoing availability, if needed, also is assured.

SUMMARY

The emotional aspects of rehabilitation are interwoven with patients' physical rehabilitation. The impact of a physical trauma, illness, or defect involves both physical and psychic components. Emotional rehabilitation is as necessary as medical or physical rehabilitation. The ways a patient deals with the stages of shock, denial, depressive reaction, reaction against independence, and adaptation will have a major role in facilitating or impeding the course of rehabilitation.

Additional aspects of the emotional impact of physical disability include the existence of previous psychiatric illness, the predisposition to traumatic losses and depression, the impact of the injury on the patient's coping strategies, the patient's place in his/her life cycle, and the effect of the residual impairment on the patient's capacity to maintain self-esteem. Emotional symptoms may include overt syndromes such as depression, anxiety, or substance abuse. They may reflect more complex issues, such as interruption in the progress of rehabilitation efforts, failure to achieve goals that are feasible, or interactional difficulties between patient, staff, families, or physicians. The negotiation of the emotional aspects of rehabilitation deserve careful attention. For some patients emotional issues are crucial in determining the benefit of all other rehabilitative efforts. The restitution of the psyche, as well as the soma, is of crucial lifelong importance. Giving up *what was* and what *might have been* allows one to see *what is* and *what can be*.

REFERENCES

Beck, A., Sethi, B. B., & Tuthill, R. W. (1963). Childhood bereavement and adult depression. *Archives of General Psychiatry, 9,* 295–302.

Brown, F. (1961). Depression and childhood bereavement. *Journal of Mental Science, 107,* 745–777.

Castelnuovo-Tedesco, P. (1981). The psychological consequences of physical trauma and defects. *International Review of Psychoanalysis, 8,* 145–154.

Greenson, R. (1967). *The technique and practice of psychoanalysis.* New York: International Universities Press.

Horowitz, M., & Kaltreider, N. (1977). Brief therapy of the stress response syndrome. *Psychiatric Clinics of North America, 2,* 356–377.

Khan, M. (1963). The concept of cumulative trauma. *The Psychoanalytic Study of the Child, 18,* 286–306.

Krueger, D. (1982). Emotional rehabilitation of the physical rehabilitation patient. *International Journal of Psychiatry in Medicine, 11,* 183–191.

Krueger, D. (1983). Childhood parent loss and adult psychopathology: Developmental considerations. *American Journal of Psychotherapy, 37,* 582–592.

Servoss, A., & Krueger, D. (1984). Normal vs. pathological grief and mourning: Some precursors. In D. Krueger (Ed.), *Emotional rehabilitation of physical trauma and disability.* (pp. 45–50) New York: Spectrum Publications.

Sethi, B. (1964). Relationship of separation to depression. *Archives of General Psychiatry, 10,* 486–496.

Steiger, H. (1976). Understanding the psychological factors in rehabilitation. *Geriatrics, 31,* 68–73.

Stewart, T. (1978). Coping behavior and the moratorium following spinal cord injury. *Paraplegia, 15,* 338–342.

Weisman, A. D. (1974). *The realization of death.* New York: Jason Aronson.

Weiss, J. (1983). *The role of narcissistic injury in medical illness.* Unpublished manuscript.

INDEX